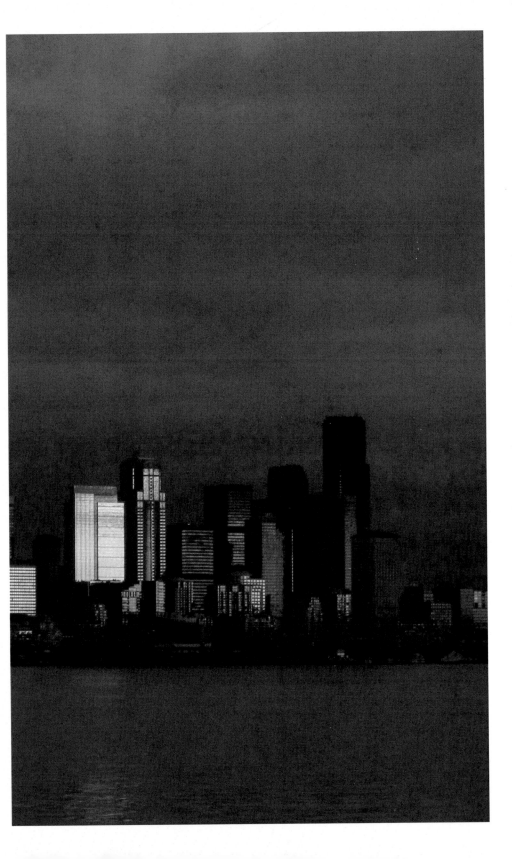

Beauty in all its sensuous forms nourishes the soul and sweeps away despair.

~Gordon Hempton, One Square Inch of Silence

What people are saying about Beating Seattle's Grey:

"An excellent summary of all the things we ALL should do daily to prevent most any ailment, not just SAD."
   —Janine Michelsons, Seattle resident

"I love this little book! Why? Because here in Seattle as anyone who has lived here knows, skies are often grey, days are short, and we often don't get enough sunshine. For some, this can lead to depression and Seasonal Affective Disorder (SAD). Beating Seattle's Grey sheds much needed light on the importance of natural daylight to our daily lives, well-being, relationships, happiness, and health. Beyond that, Beating Seattle's Grey provides a well-researched historical overview of the therapeutic effects of sunlight, and gives compelling examples from other places in the world where light deficient communities have responded effectively through good environmental design and other daylighting strategies to enhance daylight and health. It is clear that Seattleites need not continue to live and work in the dark—read the book and you will see the light!"

   —Peter Steinbrueck, Architect, FAIA

"Beating Seattle's Grey is more than a must-read for anyone living in the Pacific Northwest. In this easy-to-read guide you will learn how to live a healthier, happier life under cloudy skies."

—Gordon Hempton, Author
One Square Inch of Silence

"With Beating Seattle's Grey, Heather McAuliffe takes aim at Seattle's notorious urban winter gloom with vigor and whimsy. She diagnoses the problem and proposes tried and true solutions – along with some unconventional therapies – to break the spell of the winter blues. This richly illustrated book shines a light on a critical challenge in the built environment, and provides compelling examples of how designers, planners, and concerned citizens have sought to blunt the forces of darkness in our urban environments."

—Christopher Meek, AIA, IES
Research Associate Professor
Integrated Design Lab
UW Department of Architecture

"This book is an excellent resource - describing both the historical and modern use of natural light and exposure to the outdoors to maintain and restore good health."

—Jacqueline Bunce, DDS, MS

"Very readable and informative with great photos."

—Richard Hobday, Author
The Light Revolution

"I appreciated this book, which I found to be contemporary, uplifting, and solution-oriented!!"

—Melanie Swan, Affiliate Scholar,
Institute for Ethics and Emerging
Technologies (IEET)

"It's a wonderful book, as it put what could have been technical jargon into language and personal anecdotal experiences that I could relate to. Also, the graphs were very helpful to me as I'm a visual person and relate to bar and pie charts, and pictures!"

—Alex Rolluda, Architect, AIA

DISCLAIMER:

This book is intended to encourage readers to try out non-medical strategies to help reduce depression. It is not intended as a substitute for the medical advice of physicians. The reader should regularly consult a physician in matters relating to his/her health and particularly with respect to any symptoms that may require diagnosis or medical attention. The author is not engaged in rendering professional advice or services to the individual reader, and shall not be liable or responsible for any adverse effects or consequences that might be seen as arising from information or suggestions herein.

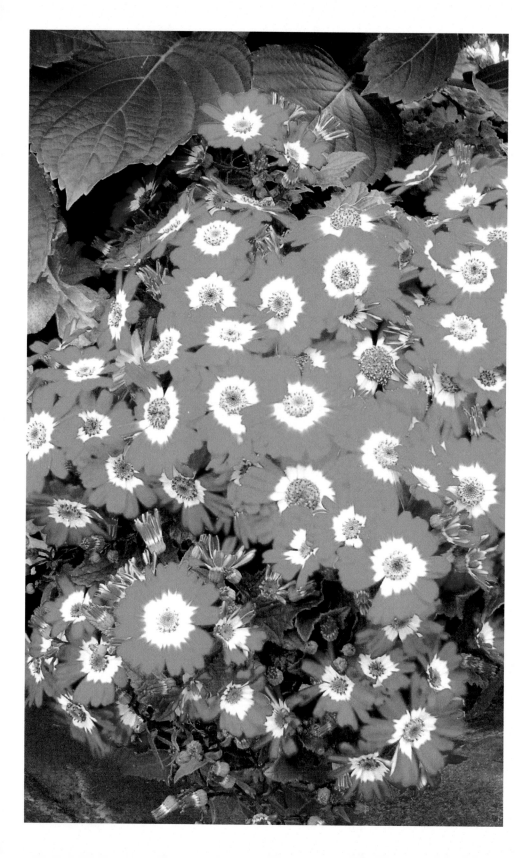

Beating
Seattle's Grey

Living in Indoor Twilight

Heather McAuliffe

Acknowledgements

I would like to thank my friends for their contributions and guidance.

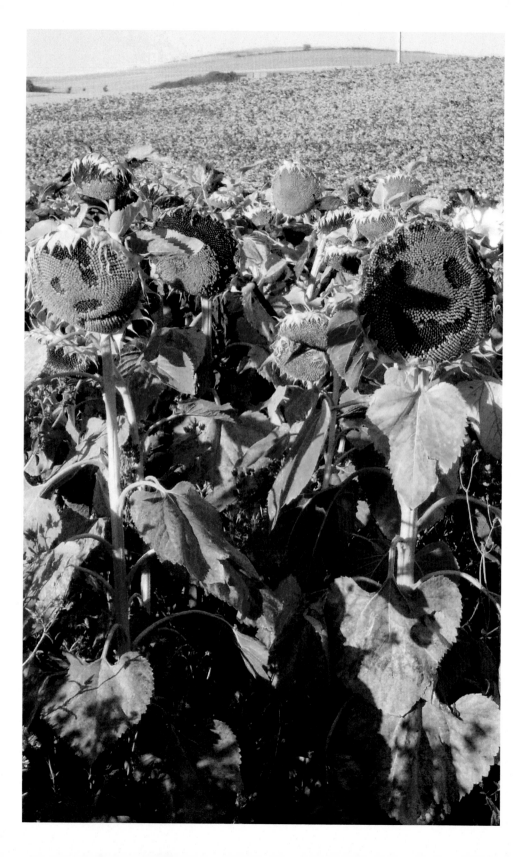

Table of Contents

-

Chapter Four
Get Some Negative Ions!

Chapter Five
Get Some Color!

"Lethargics are to be laid in the light, and exposed to the rays of the sun, for the disease is gloom."

~Arataeus, Greek physician, 6th AD.

Introduction

Seattle *is* grey. The marine weather pattern here means that it is overcast for most of the year. This means far less natural light compared to cities at lower latitudes, and also compared to inland cities that receive lots of sunshine in the summer and bright snow in the winter. The long periods of clouds and rain in Seattle are typically blamed for contributing to people here feeling depressed, i.e., less able to function, to feel motivated, and to experience joy and ease every day. When it occurs in the wintertime, this condition is called Seasonal Affective Disorder (SAD).

The lack of natural light here isn't the only potential factor in depression, however. Most of us are living a primarily indoor lifestyle. For this reason, even when it is sunny, many people in

Seattle are not exposed to enough bright light. Working almost exclusively indoors usually also means that we are spending all day inside an air conditioned environment, another factor that can contribute to the incidence of depression.

Since most of us don't have any choice but to work indoors, it is important that we learn how to mitigate the negative effects on our health from not having enough natural light and fresh air. We have to become aware of the problems, and to take action to solve them.

Beating Seattle's Grey explains how industrialization brought diseases related to sunlight deficiency and why today, after those early diseases were all but wiped out, depression persists as a major challenge to overcome. The book makes the case that depression should be blamed on our indoor lifestyle instead of Seattle's weather, and describes ways to reverse depression through awareness and making lifestyle changes. In the final chapters, the book provides suggestions for improvements to the built environment, and further research on additional factors that may contribute to depression.

Foreword

I wrote *Beating Seattle's Grey* from a compassionate viewpoint, having struggled with depression in the wintertime and successfully overcome it by using light therapy.

When I started college, my lifestyle changed drastically and I spent far less time outside. I complained about the grey, felt less motivated, and lost some of my interest and inspiration in life. I knew the grey and darkness in the winter bothered me, but I did not recognize that it was the shift in my lifestyle that had caused the shift in my attitude and mood.

After I started an office job in 1996, I became more aware of how the winter grey bothered me and recognized that I was not getting enough light. I began experimenting with artificial light therapy at home, installing daylight spectrum lights overhead, and starting light therapy with a light box. Using the light box turned out to be life-changing. I now had more energy and felt happier. Since then, many people have noticed and commented on my abundant energy and zest for life.

After experiencing the benefits of light therapy myself, I began to notice just how much the grey and indoor lifestyle affects other people. I have observed and been amazed at how much light deficiency affects all of us. I became aware that light deficiency can happen not only with the change in seasons, but also a change from an outdoor to an indoor lifestyle, or a bright workplace or home to a dark workplace or home. It is not necessarily related to the weather.

My observations and passion around the issue motivated me to want to share information on how to cope, how to overcome the problem of seasonal/lifestyle-induced depression. I began to pay more attention and think about what could be done. It became clear to me that changes to the built environment in Seattle would also help.

In 2000, I took a trip to Ireland, which has a marine climate similar to Seattle. When I visited the town of Dingle, I felt uplifted by the bright colors painted on building facades and how they contrasted with the grey skies. In comparison, Seattle has primarily drab building materials, and paint colors are typically chosen within the same palette. I was inspired by how the colors in Dingle made me feel, and have thought ever since that more color should be incorporated in Seattle at street level to enliven the pedestrian environment.

I later visited Reykjavik, another city that has marine weather patterns. I noticed how daylighting (the practice of designing to increase natural daylight) had been incorporated into buildings there, and found these spaces to be very pleasant. I thought that similar daylighting techniques could be applied in Seattle.

I have since intensively researched the causes of depression and learned about how environmental factors can contribute to it. As part of my research, I acquired meters and took measurements of light, barometric pressure, air ions and air pollution. Taking measurements on my own helped me to become more aware of the conditions in my immediate environment and to recognize changes that were happening.

I think the time has come when we should be openly discussing depression as a public health problem in Seattle and what to do about it as individuals and as a society. The main purpose of my book is to inspire people living and working in Seattle to take a closer look at their lifestyles to see what they can change in order to feel happier and have more energy, all year. It is also my goal to inspire Seattle architects and planners to improve our built environment so that all people have access to abundant light, fresh air, and color. And finally, I hope to encourage study of additional environmental factors that could be contributing to this public health problem, depression.

Heather McAuliffe

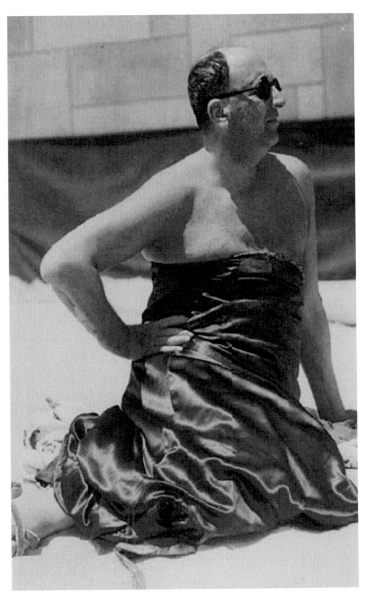

Baron Maurice de Rothchild, a member of the French Senate, enjoys a sun bath in California, 1934.

Chapter One

The Role of Sunlight

Industrialization interrupted our natural rhythms, resulting in illness

Until the industrial revolution, most people worked outside. For example, my ancestors worked in fishing and agriculture during the 1800s and the early 1900s. Their livelihoods dictated an outdoor lifestyle and their work routines were driven by the seasons.

Prior to industrialization, the amount of daylight determined when people woke up and when they went to bed. They did not use alarm clocks, and there were no indoor lights or streetlights to provide illumination throughout the night. They spent most of the day outside during the light hours, and adjusted their work routines each season as the light increased and decreased. These routines and rhythms were all changed by industrialization.

Electric lights changed this way of being in the world. People didn't need to rely on daylight anymore and were freed from the constraints of seasonal and daily darkness.

Artificial lighting brought new opportunities to expand work production. Employers could set working hours so that people were controlled by the clock. This in turn affected people's waking and sleep schedules. Instead of awakening at sunrise, it became important to use an alarm clock, in order to get up early to go to work.

Industrialization brought other questionable side effects to progress also; taller buildings shaded streets, air pollution obscured sunlight in industrial spaces. This diminution of sunlight led to new industrial illnesses in cities and urban residents suffered from high incidences of rickets and tuberculosis (TB). Before the advent of Vitamin D and antibiotics, exposure to sun and fresh air were the only known cures for these serious health problems.

The next sections in this chapter explain how tuberculosis and rickets were treated naturally at sanatoria, including in Seattle.

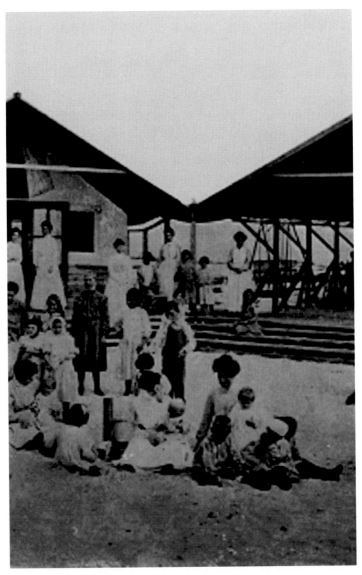

Until the advent of antibiotics, children who had tuberculosis were taken to the beach for fresh air and sunshine to help them recover. Sea Breeze Hospital, New York, c. 1900-1920.

Dr. Rollier's alpine sun treatments

The role of sunlight in alleviating skin, bone and respiratory diseases is well documented; ultraviolet light kills TB bacteria. Dr. Auguste Rollier began using sunlight in 1903 to treat TB and rickets at his alpine clinic in Switzerland. A decade later, his success had become known worldwide and it led to the popularization of sunlight treatment in the United States.

Rollier took advantage of the increased ultraviolet light high in the Swiss Alps to treat not only tuberculosis and rickets, but also smallpox and injuries. His treatment focused on exposure to the sun and a nutritious diet.

In the United States during the early 1900s, many people went to Arizona for treatment in the sunshine and dry desert. By 1920, 7,000 people had traveled to Tucson to treat tuberculosis.

By the 1930s, the use of sunlight had expanded to treat many diseases. But change, partly due to industrialization, was on the horizon: drugs replaced sunlight treatment by the 1950s.

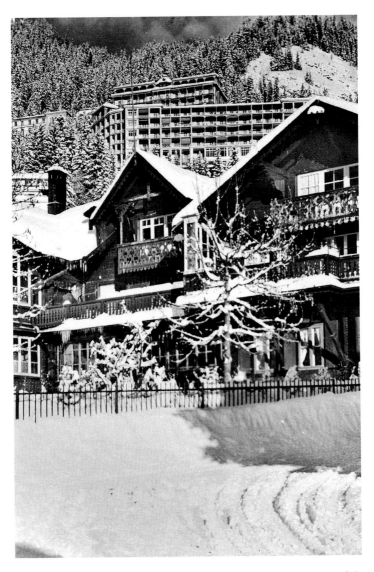

Dr. August Rollier's first sunlight treatment center opened in 1903 in Leysin, Switzerland. Patients were rolled on gurneys onto the balconies each morning, with sun exposure time gradually increased each day.

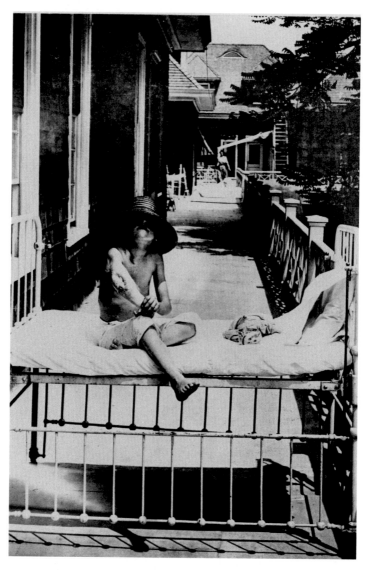

Dr. Rollier's strategy for treating tubercular and pre-tubercular patients with sunlight spread to the United States. In this photo, a young girl is exposed to sun on a balcony at Sea Breeze Hospital in New York sometime between 1900 and 1920.

Tuberculosis treatment in early Seattle

In 1908, Seattle had one of the highest rates of tuberculosis in the nation. It was the leading cause of death here, killing over 300 people each year. There were debates over where to locate a tuberculosis sanatorium in Seattle. A local doctor suggested treating the afflicted in an atrium that could be built on top of City Hall. There was an initial plan to locate a sanatorium on the west side of Queen Anne hill, but public outcry over concerns about the contagiousness of the disease stopped the plan.

Finally, the Anti-Tuberculosis League of King County was able to start a sanatorium 12 miles north of Seattle's boundary, in 1911. The new facility, Firland Sanatorium, was started with a generous donation from the League's president, Horace Henry, and half the proceeds from the Alaskan Yukon Exposition.

The sanatorium included a hospital, open air cottages, and a children's hospital with balconies for sun exposure, such as were used at Dr. Rollier's clinics in Switzerland.

HAS NEW PLAN TO FIGHT WHITE PLAGUE

Dr. W. McDowell Urges Use of Roof of New Municipal Building Where Patients Can Be Treated Under Glass.

FAULTS OF OUT-DOOR TREATMENT OVERCOME

Local Physician Believes Scheme to Place Victims in Tents Has Objections, and Suggests a Novel Idea.

IT is the belief of Dr. W. McDowell, a physician in the Crown Building, that the municipal corporation of Seattle could very properly and profitably construct a solarium on top of the new municipal building on Yesler Way where incipient cases of tuberculosis, especially where the patients are indigent, could be treated scientifically.

It is Dr. McDowell's idea that the solarium could be enclosed on at least two sides with glass and with a glass roof and open at the other sides so that there would be a complete circulation of fresh air which would be warmed to a safe temperature from the floor of the solarium, under which would be laid steam pipes.

"In suggesting the establishment of a solarium," said Dr. McDowell, "I was actuated by the consideration that the so-called outdoor treatment in many cases is not efficacious, owing to the fact that it is difficult for victims of tuberculosis to keep their underclothing dry.

"The perspiration from the body of tubercular patients is a factor to be figured on and where they live, outdoors, it is difficult to keep them comfortable and safely warm on account of this fact. It has occurred to me that by having the patients in a glass-covered room outdoors, opened on one or two sides, sufficiently above the street level to be out of the way and with a constant source of heat coming from beneath the floor, as suggested in this case, the difficulty mentioned could be overcome.

"The perspiration from a tubercular patient poisons him. On top of the municipal building there would be a large area which could be profitably used for the purposes I have outlined, the initial cost of which would be probably not to exceed $5,000.

"The patients could be supplied with rich and fattening foods and they could have all the benefit of the out-of-door treatment now so much in vogue and which has been urged as a public matter for the benefit of Seattle."

Dr. McDowell in Seattle had the idea to treat tuberculosis in an atrium on top of City Hall. Seattle Daily Times, March 30, 1908.

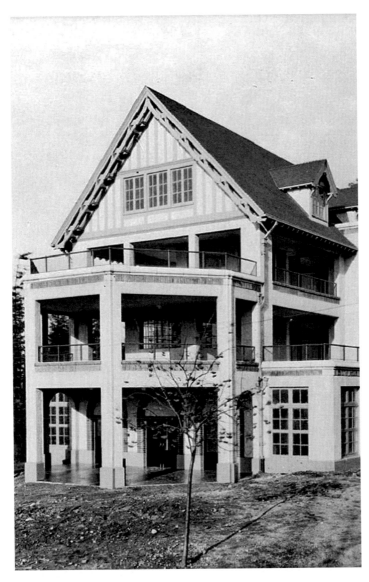

The children's hospital at Firland Sanatorium included balconies for sun exposure, much like Dr. Rollier's facilities in Switzerland.

From sunbathing to sunscreened

In the first half of the 20th century, more people worked indoors but they had also begun to sunbathe, now that the health benefits of sun and fresh air had been well publicized.

Attitudes toward tanning were also changing. In the 1890s, pale skin was considered desirable and people bathed fully clothed. But by the 1920s, they were exposing more of their skin at the beach. California and Florida became year-round destinations for a sunny vacation.

By the 1940s, people stopped using umbrellas at the beach and tanning had become especially popular. However, skin cancer showed up in the 1960s and soon doctors were cautioning people to use sunscreen to prevent overexposure.

Today, doctors continue to caution on overexposure to the sun, yet the indoor lifestyle is contributing to a deficiency in Vitamin D and rickets has reappeared as a health problem in children in the United States. How much sun is enough? How much is too much? It is a topic of continuing research and debate.

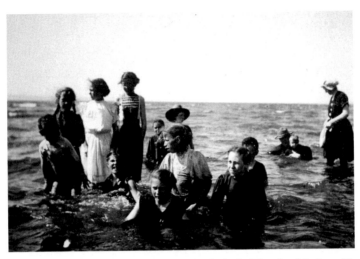

In the 1890s, people swam fully clothed. The health benefits from the sun were not yet understood. Photo taken at Ballard Beach (now Golden Gardens).

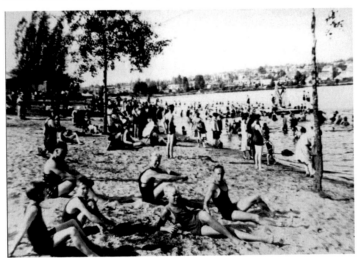

By the 20s, however, it was considered healthy to uncover more to get sun exposure. This photo shows people sunning at Green Lake's west beach in the 1920s.

About Vitamin D

By the 1920s, American doctors were aware of the importance of getting enough sunlight to prevent rickets. They educated parents about the fact that sunlight was impoverished in temperate zones and cautioned that the over-swaddling of babies could do them harm. At about the same time, research conducted on the Inuits indicated that they did not develop rickets due to their fatty fish diet. Scientists determined that it was the Vitamin D in the oil that prevented rickets. Soon, supplementing the diet with cod liver oil had all but replaced the advice to get more sun.

Since 1933, Vitamin D has been added to milk as a solution to prevent rickets. The addition of Vitamin D to the diet, however, did not expand much beyond the milk industry. Here's why: In the 1930s and 1940s, scientists experimented with extremely high dosages of Vitamin D, killing some people and permanently injuring others, due to high levels of calcium in their blood. Between the 1930s and 1990s, Vitamin D experimentation was curtailed. Then, in 1999, a Canadian researcher (Reinhold Vieth) reviewed all the toxicology studies from those years and

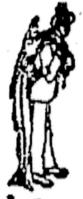
Ad for cod liver oil in the Seattle Daily Times, March 5, 1922. By the early 1920s, scientists had determined that Vitamin D in cod liver oil prevented rickets. In the 1930s, Vitamin D was added to milk.

identified differences between treating with lower and megadoses of Vitamin D. This led to a steady stream of research on Vitamin D.

Now it is understood that low Vitamin D is linked to many diseases, including but not limited to cancer, heart disease, infections, multiple sclerosis, Parkinson's and *depression.*

Work moves indoors in Seattle

Seattle's earliest industries included farming, logging and fishing. People worked outdoors all day, which meant plenty of access to sun and natural light.

World War I brought a boom in shipbuilding, so now more people started to work inside. This indoor work lifestyle was further perpetuated by another boom, this time in airplane building, during World War II.

Early warehouse buildings in Seattle were commonly built with skylights and large operable windows to provide ample light and fresh air for workers. Over the next few decades, however, building designs changed and artificial lighting and ventilation were added. Access to

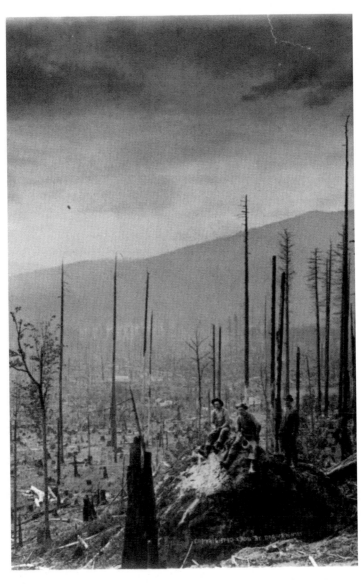

Early employment in Seattle included logging, farming and fishing. Most people worked outside and had ample access to natural light and fresh air. Logging near the Cascades, 1906.

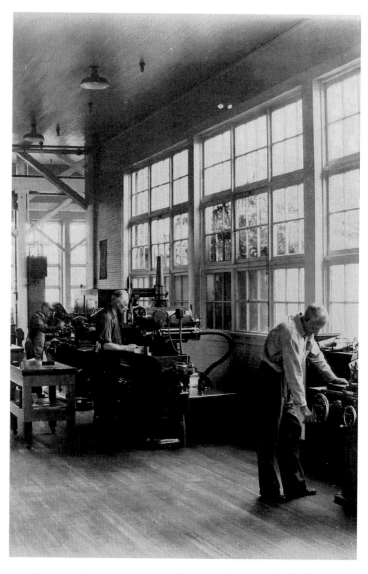

In the 1920s, access to light and fresh air was understood to be part of good health. Warehouses were constructed with large operable windows. Ivanoff Machine Shop (now Kvichak Marine Industries) in Fremont, 1920s.

natural light and fresh air were no longer considered as important.

By the 1950s, Seattle had moved well beyond the outdoor lifestyle of frontier days. Increasingly, people spent all day inside offices. Some employees now sat some distance from the nearest window, such as shown in the photos on the following pages. People were not necessarily aware of what was being sacrificed in adapting to this new indoor lifestyle that was part of industrialization in the United States.

Decades later, we are still learning about the downsides of this shift to living almost exclusively indoors. Although the diseases related to sunlight deficiency have been largely been eradicated, many people now suffer instead from an insidious condition related to *light deficiency:* depression.

The next chapter explains why the shift to an indoor lifestyle (and indoor lighting), instead of Seattle's grey weather, may be to blame for Seasonal Affective Disorder in Seattle.

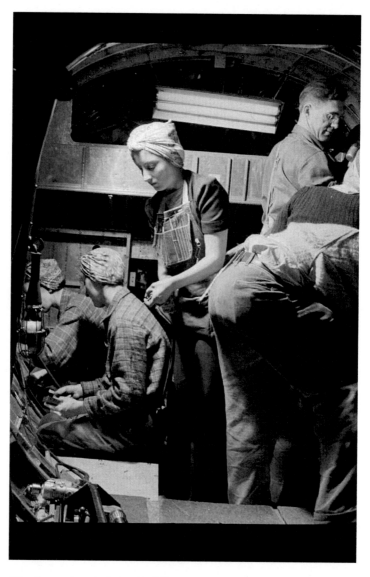

The boom in airplane building during World War II brought many indoor jobs. In this 1942 photo of workers at Boeing, their only source of light is a set of fluorescent light bulbs.

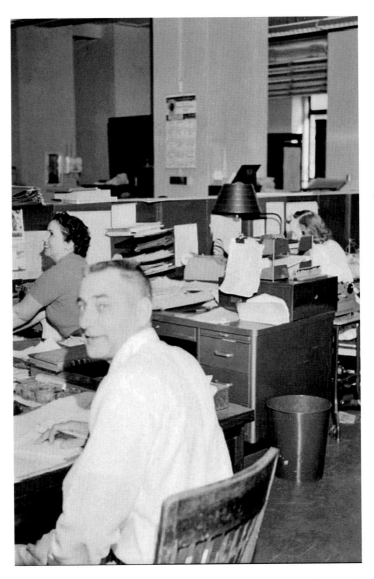

By the 1950s, office work was more common, with people working inside away from the windows, such as at the Street Use and Permits Section office (City of Seattle) pictured above.

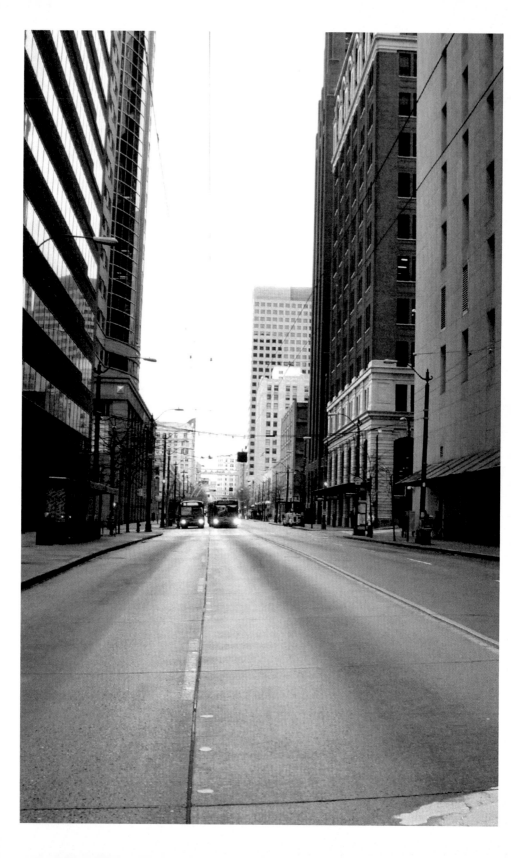

Chapter Two

About Seattle's Grey

Seattle's location, weather and winter

Seattle can be very grey, downright dark in the winter. Its location at just over 47 degrees north of the equator means short winter days. The marine weather and the mountain ranges on either side of Puget Sound bring long periods of cloud cover that limit the light even more.

Seattle has clear or partially cloudy days only *four to eight days* each month in the winter, according to the Western Regional Climate Center. And, since the start of Daylight Savings Time was shifted two weeks earlier in 2007, we have dark mornings into April. All this darkness can make it difficult to get up and going!

The long overcast periods and short days are frequently blamed for affecting people's moods.

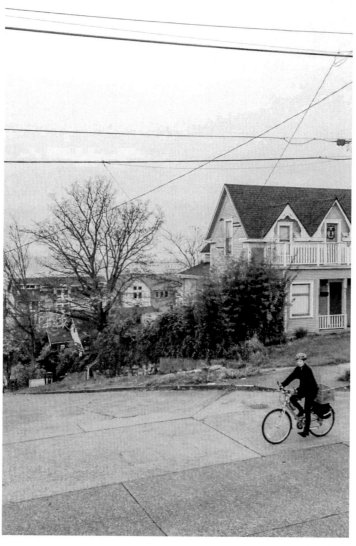

Seattle has only four to eight clear (or partially cloudy) days each month in the winter. This makes for long overcast periods.

The winter becomes a time when some people respond to the darkness like hibernating bears, staying indoors most of the time. This chapter explains how too little light affects us, and why Seattle's weather and short winter days probably are not the main reasons why people get Seasonal Affective Disorder here.

Light levels at noon: one year in Seattle

I was aware that we have less light in the winter and lots more in the summer, but I was interested in knowing *exactly* how much light we receive each season. For that reason, I bought a light meter and took measurements at noon for a year, both outdoors and indoors.

The graphs on the following pages provide the results of my measurements outdoors in *lux*, a unit for measuring illuminance (available light). I tracked the light levels outside in the same place each day at noon, with the sensor held vertically to simulate the experience of a person who is standing, walking or sitting. The results are not surprising; they show lots of brighter days in spring and summer, with progressively fewer in the autumn and winter.

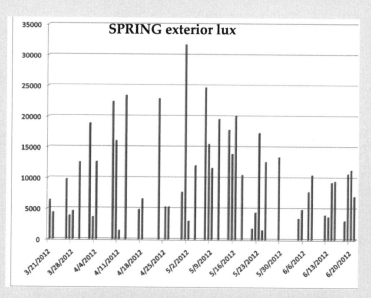

Spring exterior lux measurements. Average: 10,000 lux.

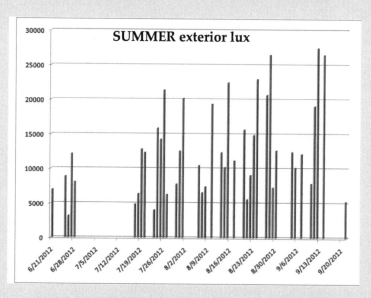

Summer exterior lux measurements. Average: 13,000 lux.

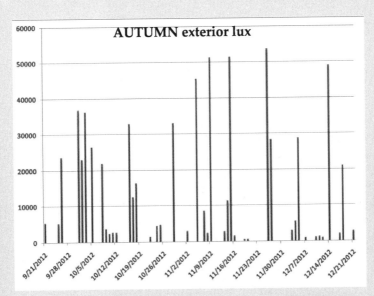

Autumn exterior lux measurements. Average: 16,000 lux.

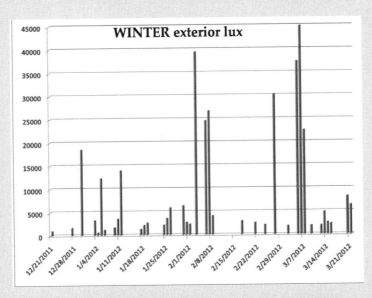

Winter exterior lux measurements. Average: 10,000 lux.

The graph of winter measurements shows lots of dim days, but also a number of sunny days that were incredibly bright at noon (at eye level), due to the position of the sun in the winter. When these much higher measurements were included, the average daily illuminance was raised to 10,000 lux, the equivalent of a *standard therapeutic light box*. Moreover, there were many days when the illuminance was at least 2500 lux, the minimum required to reset our body clock (more on this in Chapter Three). This is great news, because it means that Seattle's grey doesn't matter so much!

The results led me to believe that if we just spent more time outside in the winter, we would be less likely to get SAD. But here is the problem: Now that most people are staying indoors all day, the amount of illuminance outdoors doesn't matter so much anymore.

Since living and working indoors means being exposed to artificial light all day, it would seem important to find out how the illuminance indoors compares to the illuminance outside. For that reason, I decided to measure indoor illuminance six feet from a window for a year.

The results are graphed on the next two pages. I found that the average illuminance was 300-400 lux, regardless of the time of year. This is less than the illuminance I measured outdoors (at noon) on the dimmest days in January. Until I took measurements myself, I didn't realize just how dark it was indoors!

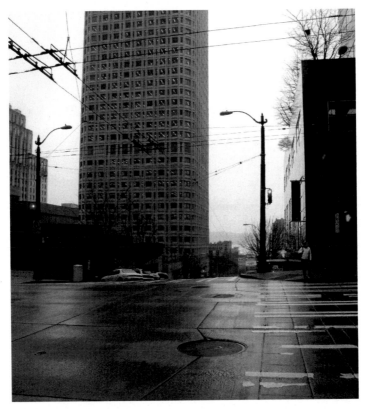

*In measuring indoor illuminance six feet from a window, I was surprised to find that it was consistently less than illuminance outside on our darkest days in the wintertime. Above: **450 lux**.*

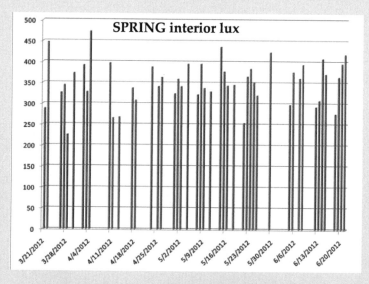

*Spring interior lux measurements. Average: **350 lux**.*

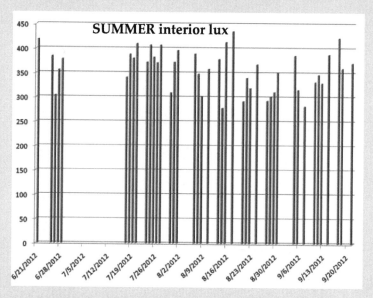

*Summer interior lux measurements. Average: **350 lux**.*

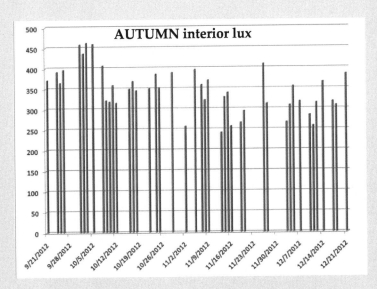

*Autumn interior lux measurements. Average: **400 lux**.*

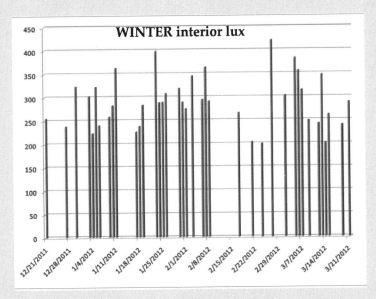

*Winter interior lux measurements. Average: **300 lux**.*

Living in an indoor twilight

Richard Hobday makes the case in his book, *The Light Revolution: Health, Architecture and the Sun,* that staying indoors all day is equivalent to living in twilight. He bases this on the fact that typical indoor illuminance, 50-500 lux, is the same as the illuminance at twilight, when the sun has just dropped below the horizon on a summer evening.

Today most people work in indoor occupations and the only natural light they get outdoors is during a few minutes at lunchtime. In winter, many leave before sunrise and return home after dark.

People who work primarily indoors can be depressed from light deficiency without being aware of the problem. The symptoms come on gradually and then it becomes a way of life, just a way to be. If we are spending most of our time indoors *all year,* it is possible to suffer depression from light deficiency not only in the winter (SAD), but also during the rest of the year. A list of symptoms related to light deficiency follows the photos on the next page.

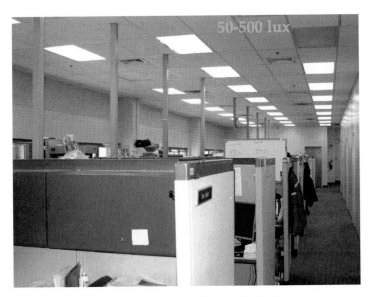

Illuminance at most offices: 50-500 lux.

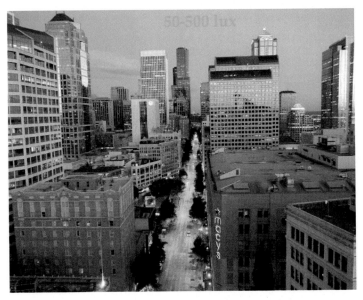

Illuminance at twilight in the summer: 50-500 lux.

Light deficiency symptoms

The first symptoms of lack of light can be:

- Feeling tired and less energetic
- Being in a bad mood
- Difficulty concentrating
- Headache
- Little or no desire to go outside or be active

Continued light deficiency can lead to:

- Sleep disorders
- Increased appetite and weight gain
- Depressed immune system
- Decreased sex drive
- Declining social life

Source: A Life In Lux: Bright Insights About Wellness
Hippas Eriksson

Since it appears that the consistently dim lighting indoors is to blame for our problems related to light deficiency, it would make sense to focus on changing our lifestyles to get enough light each day.

Spending more time outdoors would be an obvious solution. However, some people are not able to get outside long enough on short winter days due to work and other demands on their daily schedules. This can lead to light deficiency symptoms and related health problems. Being aware of these issues can motivate us to make lifestyle adjustments in order to feel better.

The next chapter offers some creative strategies for adding more light to our daily routines. When we have access to enough bright light, we can more easily achieve a positive mood and live with more energy in spite of spending the day time indoors in poorly lit spaces.

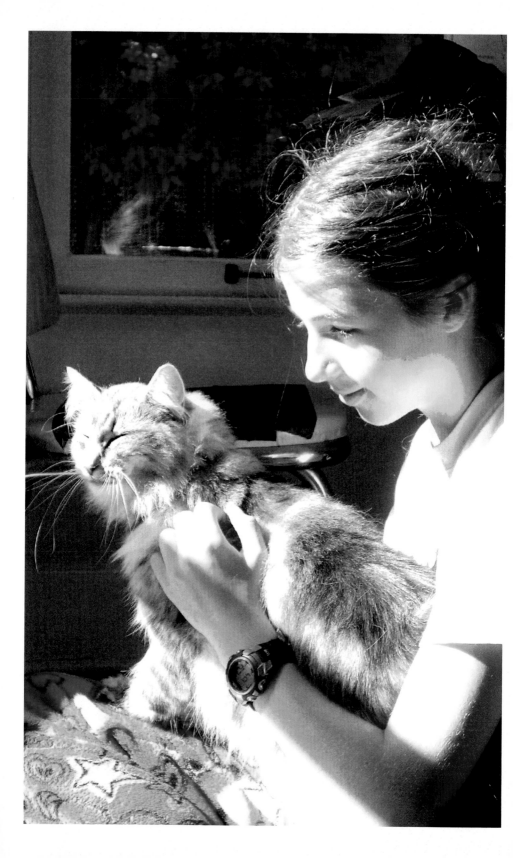

Chapter Three

Get Some Light!

We need bright light in the morning

Bright light in the morning is essential to wake us up, to shut off the production of the sleep hormone (melatonin) and to enable the production of the 'happiness hormone' (serotonin). If the production of melatonin is not shut down, then it competes with the production of serotonin. This can leave us feeling sleepy and lethargic, and make it more difficult to be in a good mood.

Social jet lag makes us out of sync

According to sleep researchers at the University of Munich, waking early during the weekdays and sleeping in on the weekends causes "social jet lag," a condition in which our circadian rhythms are out of sync with our schedules. Although most of the attention from the research

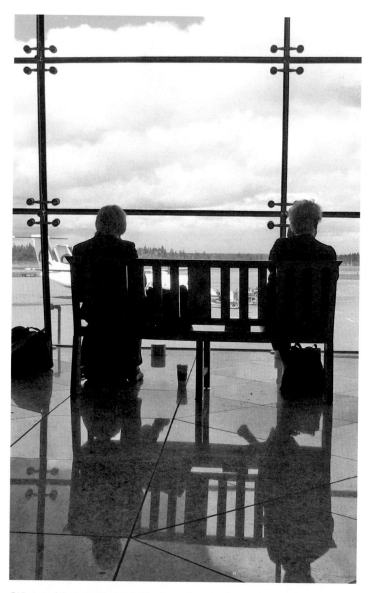

We need bright light daily in order to shut off the production of the sleep hormone and to enable the production of the 'feel good' hormone. At least 2500 lux is necessary to reverse SAD.

has been on the link to obesity, switching waking time back and forth has also been implicated as a risk factor for developing depression. The changing in waking time on Monday can affect a person's mood and energy level for several days.

Social jet lag is becoming more of a problem than ever, according to sleep scientists. They explained that it is thus: people are spending less time outside; this resets their body clock so that they are awake later at night. Fortunately, social jet lag, just like SAD, can be reversed with enough light in the morning.

Evening types ("night owls") may be more prone to social jet lag. The tendency toward eveningness (staying up late) may actually be a result of insufficient exposure to daytime light, studies have suggested.

A 2002 Japanese study of junior high students indicated that the students who went outside during class breaks and lunch were more likely to be morning types.

Kenneth Wright, a neuroscientist and chronobiology expert at the University of

Boulder, found that he could change sleeping and waking times of night owls to an earlier schedule just by exposing them to natural light-dark cycle during a weeklong camping trip.

The phenomenon of eveningness/morningness is currently being researched intensively around the world because of its great impact to health.

Low morning light can affect our weight

Morning light sets circadian rhythms, including metabolism. A recent study indicated that those who were exposed to bright light before noon generally speaking, lighter in weight even when exercise, diet and sleep were taken into account.

It is not clear how light helps people stay trimmer but it does affect metabolism and reduces feelings of hunger and satiety. It is clear that light has many benefits beyond alertness.

About light therapy

The earliest studies on light therapy conducted in the 1980s by the National Institutes of Health determined that we need exposure to at least 2500 lux of light to reverse the symptoms of SAD. These findings have since been updated to advise the use of 10,000 lux as a standard for light therapy. 10,000 lux is roughly equivalent to the light we would receive outside in April.

If people are indoors all day, they are generally exposed to only **50-500** lux all the time. That is really low! Even if they sit next to a window, it may not be enough. As shown in the photos on the next page, it would be necessary have to have one's nose pressed up against the window to get the benefit of the light coming through the window.

If people are indoors all day, they are generally exposed to only 50-500 lux all the time. That is really low!

If we are working indoors in Seattle, getting enough light becomes very challenging in the winter. Any light beyond what we receive indoors would still an improvement. Although it is unlikely that we can find 10,000 lux on dark mornings in the winter here (without using a light box), there are some great ways to get more light at lunchtime.

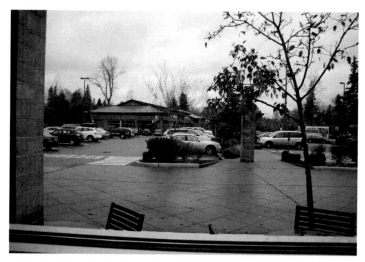

In late November, facing out a north facing window (2' away): 1215 lux. Okay, but still pretty low. To do better, one's nose really would have to be pressed up against the window.

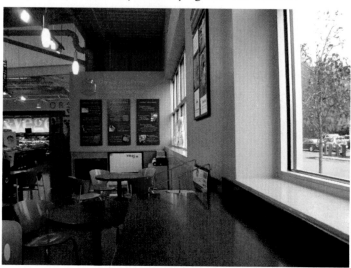

Facing alongside the same window: 350 lux. This is really low. Typically when people position theirs desks near windows, it is alongside. They may not be getting enough light!

Sun breaks

Sunny days are fewer in the winter, but they offer an excellent opportunity to get a huge dose of light in just a short time. In my research, I measured illuminance in sunny spots around Seattle at noon in January from 80,000 to 120,000 lux, 8-12 times the illuminance of a therapeutic light box.

Because of its position low in the sky during the winter, the sun's illuminance at noon (at eye level) is about three times greater than at noon in the summer. The sun can be a powerful light box at lunchtime!

In the winter, sunny spots at noon in Seattle can provide 8-12 times the illuminance of a therapeutic light box.

Since indoor lighting is usually insufficient for our body's daily needs, it would make sense to deliberately take sun breaks whenever the sun is out in the winter. Standing or walking in sunny areas could recharge the mood and energy level. When the sun is so bright, it does not take long.

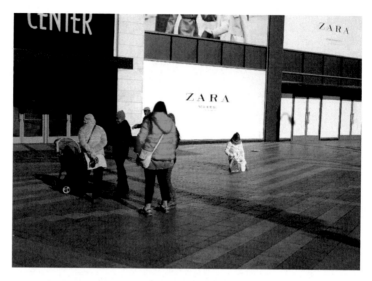

Illuminance at Westlake Plaza in February at noon: 120,000 lux.

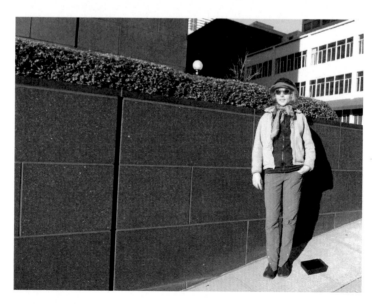

Illuminance at 5th & Marion in December at noon: 82,000 lux.

Despite the increasing number of tall buildings in downtown Seattle, there are still lots of public places where it is possible to find bright spots whenever the sun comes out in the winter. Thanks to legislation championed by Seattle City Councilmember Peter Steinbrueck in 2007 that called for surveying historic buildings downtown, and successful preservation efforts, today there remain shorter buildings in the downtown core that preserve sunlit areas not blocked by taller structures.

Below are examples of some locations that receive intense sun in downtown Seattle at noon in the winter. Adding a 15-minute sun break at lunch would help improve the health and outlook of people who work in downtown Seattle.

15-minute sun breaks at noon in winter, downtown Seattle

- 1st Avenue, east side: Marion to Virginia
- 1st & Marion: Fed. Building public terraces
- 2nd & Spring: NE corner
- 2nd & University: Symphony Hall plaza
- 4th & Cherry: NW corner
- 4th Avenue, east side, Columbia to Madison

- 4th & Madison: Fourth & Madison Building, 7th floor plaza (Podium elevators)
- 4th & Madison, NE corner, library plaza
- 4th & Pine: Westlake Plaza
- 5th & Columbia, NE corner: BofA plaza
- 5th & James: Muni Court plaza
- 5th & King: 505 Union plaza
- 5th & Marion: NE corner and north side
- 5th & Spring: U.S. Court of Appeals lawn
- 6th & Union: One & Two Union Sq. plazas
- Cherry St: between 3rd and 4th, north side
- Columbia: between 1st and 2nd, north side
- Columbia: between 4th and 5th, north side
- Madison: between 1st and 2nd, north side
- Pike Place Market
- Seattle waterfront and Sculpture Park

Indoor atria for light

When the sun isn't out in the winter, it is still possible to get some added natural light at lunchtime. Although not as bright as a sunny day, public atria provide significantly more illuminance than found inside most buildings.

I measured lux levels in some atria in downtown Seattle. I found that the illuminance was *four to eight* times the average I had measured indoors.

Spending time daily outside or in an atrium can help to meet our bodies' needs for light. Photos of some atria in Seattle are included below and on the following pages.

Indoor atria in downtown Seattle

- 1st & Pike: Economy Market atrium
- 3rd & Seneca: Chase Center atria
- 4th & Pine: Westlake Mall food court
- 5th & Pine: U.S. Bank atrium
- 5th & Spring: Downtown Library - 10th floor
- 6th & Pine: Pacific Place atrium
- 8th & Pike: Washington State Convention Center atria

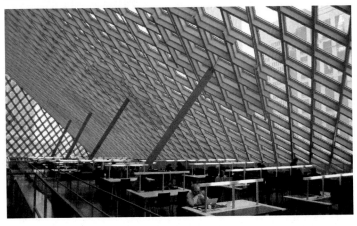

The tenth floor atrium at the downtown branch of the Seattle Public Library provides daylit space for quiet activities.

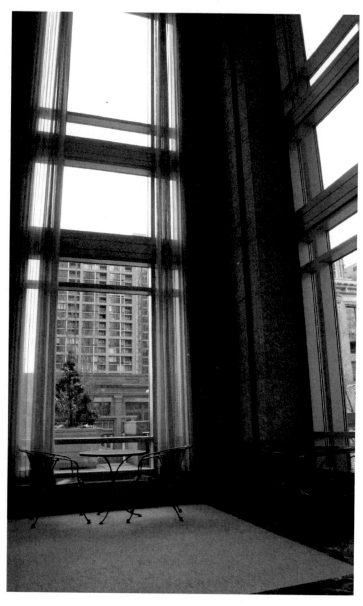

The Chase Center atrium at 3rd & Seneca is divided into three sections. The tall windows create pleasant daylit space.

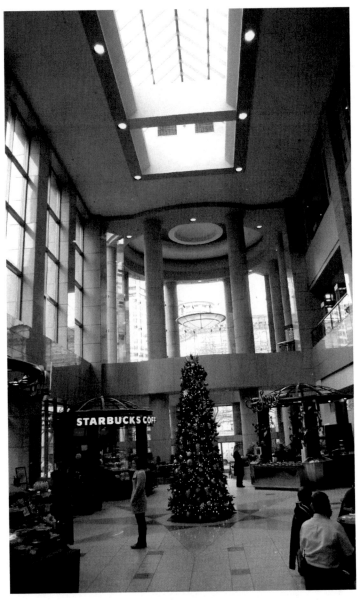

Tall windows and a large skylight make the US Bank lobby atrium at 5th & Pine a pleasant daylit gathering space.

81

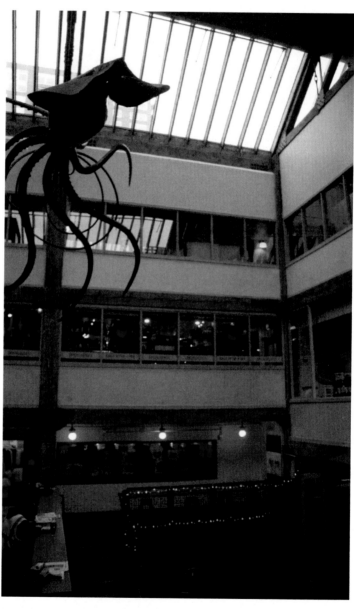

At 1st and Pike, the Economy Atrium (Pike Place Market) is daylit by an enormous skylight.

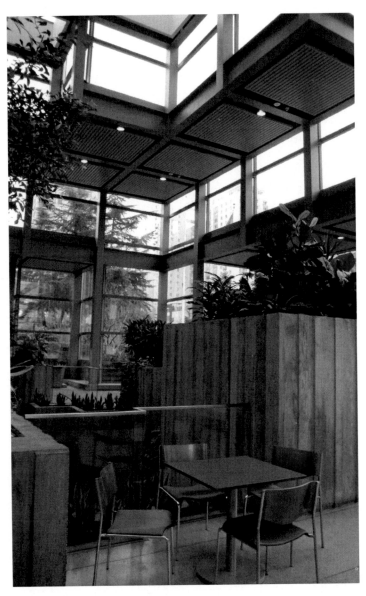

The public atrium at the Washington State Convention Center (8th and Pike) features natural light and plants.

83

Privately Owned Public Spaces (POPS)

In addition to public areas, there are privately owned public spaces (POPS) in downtown Seattle, some indoors and some outdoors. Many of them offer great natural light, such as the plaza shown on the next page. These spaces are usually marked with a sign informing the public that it is public space. For more information and a map, visit www.seattle gov/DPD .

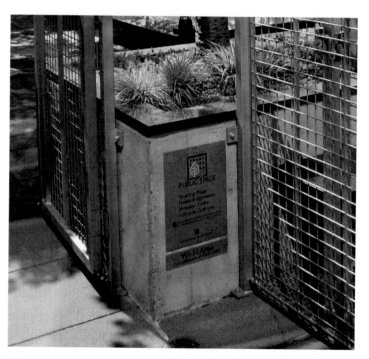

Private property designated as public space is marked with a sign that explains that it is public space.

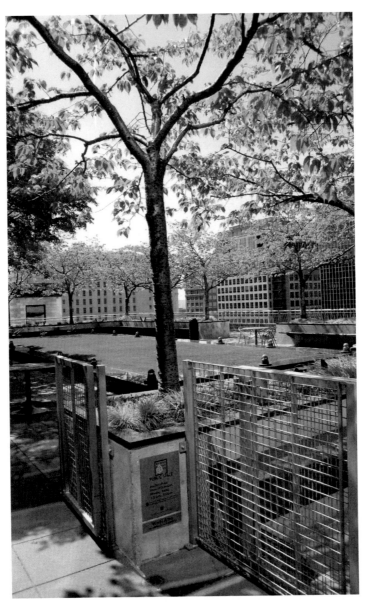

The designated public space at the Fourth & Madison Building (7th Floor Plaza), provides an urban oasis on sunny days.

85

What we wear, how we travel, may keep us in the dark

For people who spend all day indoors, the choices that they make when they go outside in the daytime can affect whether or not they are getting enough light overall. In the winter, it is important to allow the light outdoors to reach our eyes. If we don't receive the light, then our bodies continue to produce melatonin, leaving us sleepy and lethargic.

• Hoods and brimmed hats can limit light coming into the eyes, particularly on a grey day.

• Sunglasses block most of the light directed into our eyes. They should not be necessary on grey days.

• Dark or opaque umbrellas block natural daylight. Transparent umbrellas allow more light through them.

• Traveling for long periods inside cars, buses and trains can limit our exposure to daylight. Walking part of the way can help increase light exposure.

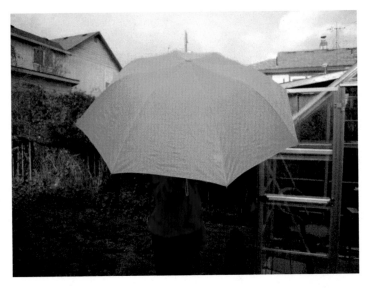

Illuminance under an opaque umbrella in January: **600 lux**

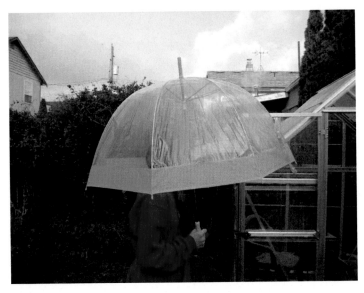

Illuminance under a transparent umbrella in January: **1200 lux**

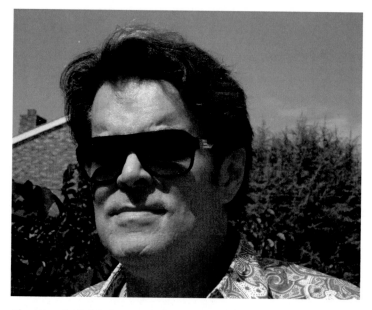

If natural light is our only source of bright light, wearing sunglasses could contribute to the problem of light deficiency.

Sunglasses and light deficiency

Sunglasses usually block at least 90% of the available illuminance. People who wear sunglasses anytime they go outside might not be getting enough light, especially if being outdoors is their only exposure to bright light. If wearing sunglasses is necessary, then artificial light therapy might help to meet the body's need for light. For people whose eyes are too sensitive to use a light box, there is an alternative light therapy available (described later in this chapter).

Add more natural daylight at home

Seattle housing styles were often copied from sunnier places around the United States, so they were not designed to maximize natural light. My house, for example, could have been copied after a farmhouse in Illinois - it has few windows relative to the amount of wall space. It can be quite dark inside, particularly in the winter. However, there are things we can do to mitigate the light-poor designs of our homes.

Drapes and blinds should be opened first thing in the morning. Furniture and plants that block the incoming light should be moved *away* from the windows. Dining tables and desks, places where we spend lots of time, should be located right next to the windows.

Skylights and an atrium can add more daylight where it is needed in the daytime. A cheaper alternative is to buy a small greenhouse and use it for people instead of plants. I bought a 4' x 6' greenhouse (see next page) and found that I could use it nearly all year due to the mild temperatures in Seattle. The heat from a hot drink is usually sufficient to warm the small structure.

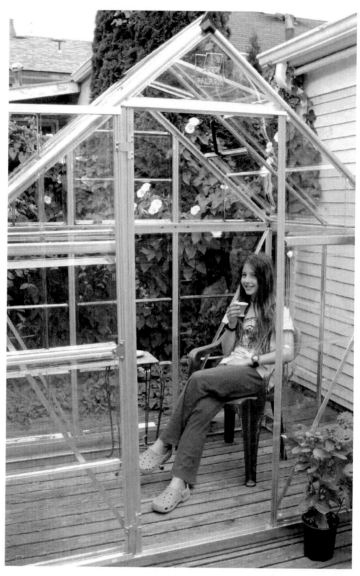

The heat from a hot drink can be sufficient to warm up this small (4' x 6') polycarbonate greenhouse on mild winter days. The structure adds a bright daylit space to a dark home.

90

Get some altitude

Ultraviolet light intensity increases 4% every 1,000 feet above sea level. For that reason, it is possible to get lots of sun in the wintertime on top of local foothills in the Cascade Mountains such as Tiger Mountain and Mount Si. Both of these popular hiking destinations are accessible by bus from Seattle.

The photo below, taken in late November at the West Tiger #3 summit of Tiger Mountain (3000 feet), shows that the sun is quite intense even though it is nearly winter.

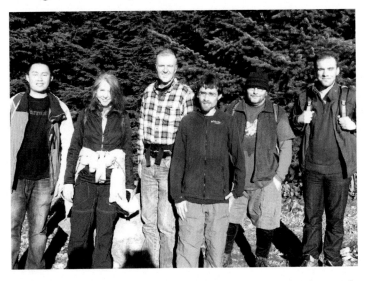

Although it is late November, the sun is very bright at the summit of Tiger Mountain (due to the altitude).

Visit a local sunny place

Some people escape for a sunny vacation every winter as a way to cope with the grey winters here. However, most of us need a more affordable alternative. One option is to visit a *local* sunny place. Within one to three hours' drive, it is possible to escape the rain, either by going east of the Cascade Mountains, or to the *rain shadow* of the Olympic Mountains.

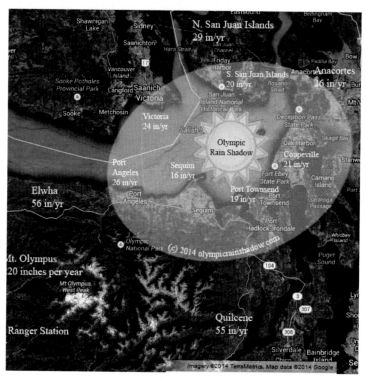

Map of Olympic Rain Shadow

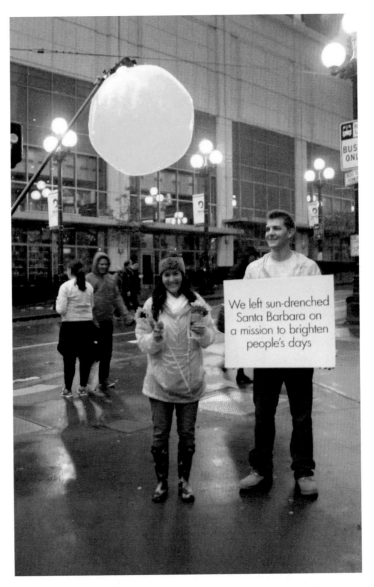

There are cheaper ways to find light in Seattle than leaving town! Santa Barbara sun emissaries promoting visits to the "American Riviera" in Seattle, November 2014.

Live or work in a sunnier neighborhood

A few years ago, I read a compelling book by local historian and walking guidebook author Harvey Manning, *Walking the Beach to Bellingham.* Mr. Manning described in his book how he was inspired to head west from his home in Cougar Mountain for a walk whenever he saw a blue hole over Seattle.

After reading the book, I started noticing that there were consistently "blue holes" over Ballard when it remained cloudy downtown. Eventually I had a chance to ask atmospheric scientists in Seattle about it. They confirmed that we do indeed have small rain shadows caused by the major hills in Seattle. The wind blows primarily from the southwest and creates rain shadows northeast of the hills.

The isometric map on the following page shows the patterns of rainfall in Seattle during the 1987-88 rainy season. The rainfall is about 40" upwind of the hills, and about 35" downwind of the hills.

If we need more light daily, it might help to live or work in a sunnier neighborhood!

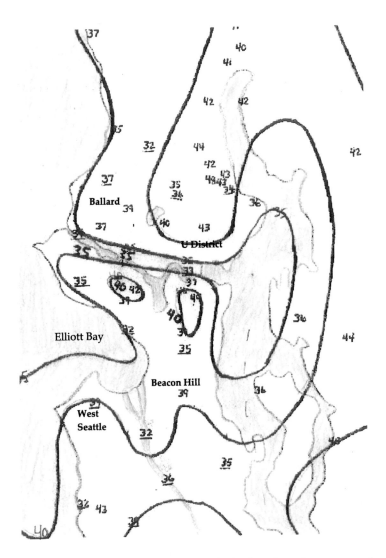

Map of small rain shadows in Seattle during the rainy season of 1987-88. The lines indicate areas of equal rainfall. The map shows that the major hills in Seattle, Beacon Hill, Magnolia, Queen Anne and Capitol Hill cast small rain shadows. Neighborhoods northeast of the hills receive less rainfall.

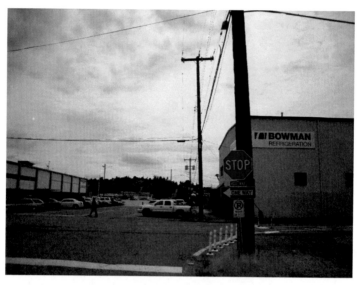

Looking south from NW 45th St. and 14th Ave NW in Ballard, the clouds cover downtown and Queen Anne.

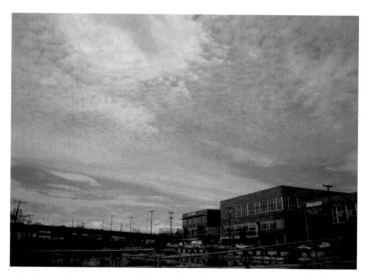

At the same time, to the west, the cloud cover is breaking up due to the rain shadow from Magnolia's hill.

Vitamin D in the winter

To make adequate Vitamin D (a hormone) ourselves, we have to directly expose our skin to sunlight. Seattle is just too far north of the equator for us to get enough sun in the winter.

Since low Vitamin D has been linked to so many diseases and conditions, including depression, it would make sense for everyone living here to get tested for Vitamin D deficiency, especially people who work indoors year round! People who have dark skin are at special risk for being deficient, because it takes more sunlight to get their skin to produce Vitamin D.

The only way to find out one's level of Vitamin D is to get a blood test. Recommendations on how much Vitamin D to take are based on the blood test results and the person's diet and exposure to sunlight. When I was working indoors fulltime, I learned that despite riding my bike daily to work and jogging several days a week, my Vitamin D level was at the low end of normal. After successfully raising the level through supplementation, I experienced a wonderful surprising outcome: I stopped catching other people's colds!

Bright light therapy works

Bright light therapy has been used successfully since the 1980s to reverse depression from light deficiency. It has become mainstreamed as a treatment, so insurance plans commonly cover it. Although it is possible to get enough light year round by going outdoors, people who work indoors all day would probably benefit from daily artificial light therapy, particularly during the wintertime. In my personal experience as an indoor worker, using a light box made a huge difference in my ability to function and enjoy life in the dark days of winter.

The standard illuminance of a therapeutic light box is 10,000 lux. Researchers have advised that the light should be tilted (as shown on the next page) to allow more light to enter the eyes while decreasing glare. The light is typically used in the morning for at least 15 minutes. It can be used during the afternoon also, but should not be used at night, since the bright light delays the production of melatonin.

For people whose eyes are too sensitive for light therapy, an alternative to light boxes is included in the next section.

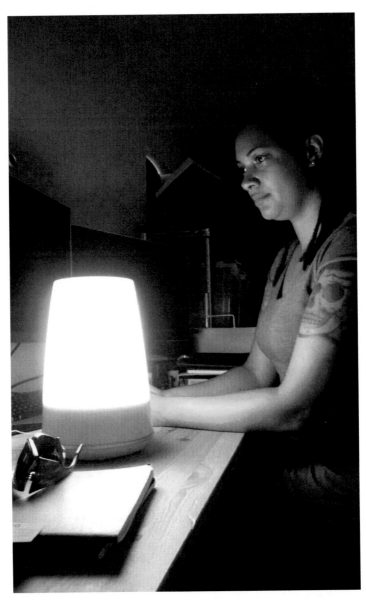

Bright light therapy has been used successfully since the 1980s to reverse depression from light deficiency.

Alternatives to light boxes

If using a light box is not convenient, there are more portable options available, such as light visors or handheld devices. Another alternative, which could work for people whose eyes are too sensitive to light, is to use light *earphones*. Valkee Oy, a company located in northern Finland, developed a device that uses LED lights to stimulate the brain where the skull is at its thinnest, inside the ears. The lights are used for 8-12 minutes in the morning to prevent SAD. They have also been found effective in preventing and reducing jet lag .

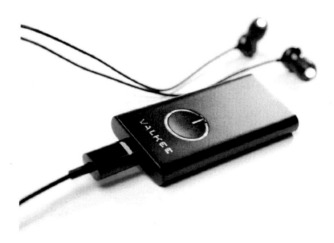

Valkee's HumanCharger® light earphones deliver blue LED light to the brain through the ear canals. Treatment time is 8-12 minutes.

A dawn simulator is another type of light therapy that has been found to help reduce wintertime depression by regulating circadian rhythms. A timer is attached to a bright light and turns on the light gradually in the morning.

How much light?

How much light we need each day is something we have to determine for ourselves. It would help to measure the daytime illuminance at home and at work, wherever we spend most of our day indoors. It is something we can easily test ourselves with a portable light meter or a light meter phone app. Another option is to wear a personal light tracker that tracks bright light exposure. Monitoring the amount of light ourselves is not only empowering, it can provide motivation to make lifestyle changes.

Reduce blue light at night

Although we need bright light during the day, we should avoid it at night, to be able sleep well. Bright blue light from computers, tablets, phones and televisions is stimulating and could make it difficult to fall and stay asleep. A 2012 study indicated that melatonin was suppressed by 22% in people using electronic devices with blue backlit displays for two hours at night. Additionally, light at night has been linked to obesity and cancer.

If it is necessary to use a computer at night, the stimulating effect from the blue light can be reduced by using software that changes the color of the screen to a warmer color after nightfall. Free software to make this change, f.lux, is available to download at www.justgetflux.com.

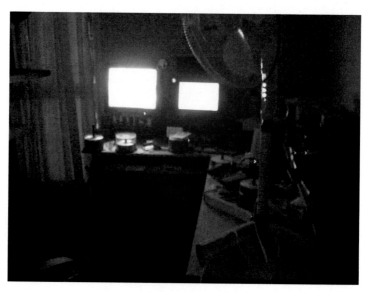

The blue light from backlit displays on electronic devices is stimulating and can make it difficult to fall and stay asleep.

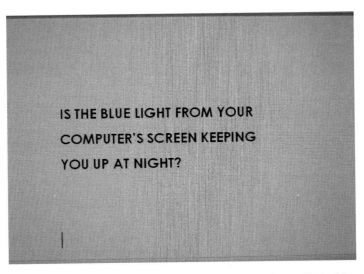

*This photo shows a computer screen with typical blue backlighting, **6500 kelvin.***

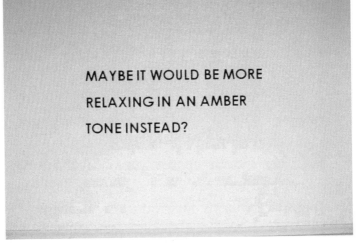

*With f.lux sofware activated at **2700 kelvin,** the screen takes on an amber tone. This color of light is less stimulating to the brain.*

103

If we are indoors all day, there are myriad ways to get more light on a daily basis. It is often just a matter of making lifestyle adjustments, such as spending time outside in the morning, lunching in an atrium and walking part of the way home; or, by adding light therapy.

People need to be aware that adequate light exposure light is a *daily bodily need* and that they have to deliberately take action to get enough light, since homes and indoor workplaces often do not offer sufficient light. Monitoring one's own light exposure is a great way to find out more about the issue, and can provide motivation to make appropriate lifestyle changes.

In addition to seeking out more light daily, there are other things we can do to help keep from getting depressed from an indoor lifestyle. The next chapter explains how fresh air therapy was historically to treat respiratory illnesses, why the air quality in indoor spaces can contribute to depression, and how we can mitigate the effects of problematic indoor and outdoor air quality through exposure to more negative ions.

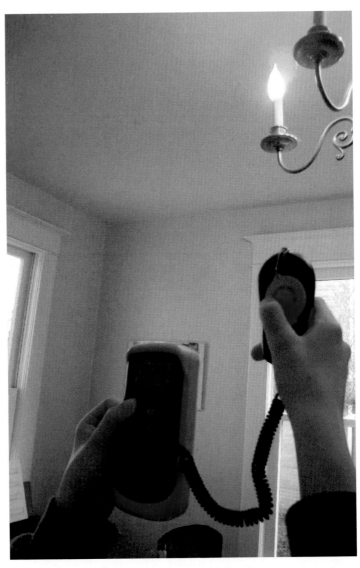

Measuring the light levels at home and work can be informative and motivate us to make changes. Even moving a desk to face a window can make quite a difference in the amount of light we receive. Sometimes it takes measuring light to figure this out!

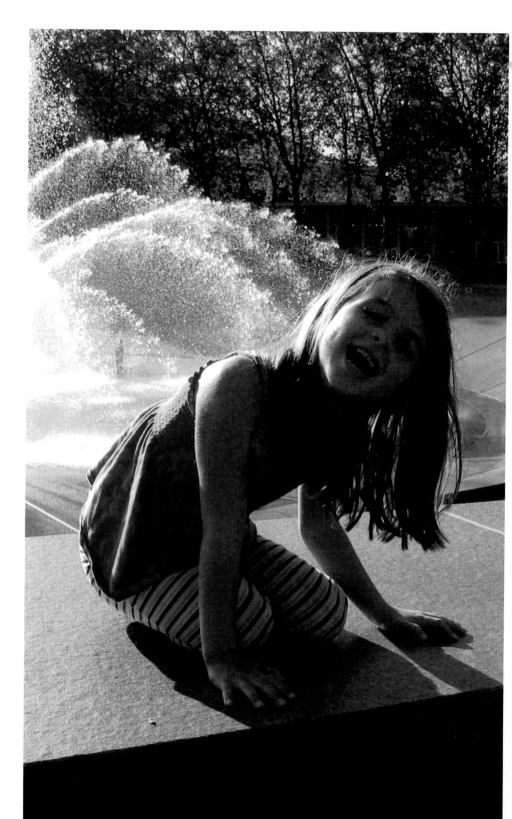

Chapter Four

Get Some Negative Ions!

Fresh air healed and prevented TB

The importance of fresh air in maintaining health was recognized early in the 20th century. Patients who suffered from tuberculosis were sent away from the cities to sanatoriums that were located in the mountains or near the sea.

Relying on fresh air as a remedy for tuberculosis also resulted in the *open air* school movement. Open air schools were developed initially as a way to prevent tuberculosis in vulnerable children and were later used to *promote mental health in physically healthy children.*

Open air schools were built with large windows and heating systems that would work while the windows were open. In the winter, children were bundled up warmly in their classrooms while the windows were left open.

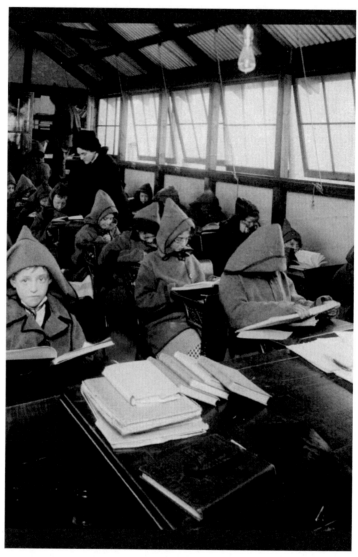

In the early 1900s, "open air schools" were built with large windows and heating systems that would work while the windows were open. Their use for tuberculosis prevention was later expanded to promote mental health in healthy children.

Seattle's early schools were designed with large windows to allow in plenty of fresh air. B.F. Day Elementary School, pictured on the next page, includes additions that were built in 1916 at the height of the open air school movement. The large center pivot type windows installed on these sections of the building maximized natural ventilation. As noted in Chapter One, early warehouse buildings in Seattle that were used for factory work also included large windows that opened to allow in lots of fresh air.

HVAC systems replaced use of windows

By the 1950s, tuberculosis had been eradicated with drugs, so natural ventilation was considered less important. Since that time, heating, ventilation and air conditioning (HVAC) systems have been added to buildings to create comfortable indoor environments. To keep these systems energy efficient, windows are no longer allowed to be used or do not open, such as in hermetically sealed office towers. Although HVAC systems can ventilate closed spaces in place of windows, they do not provide much fresh air. This is a problem!

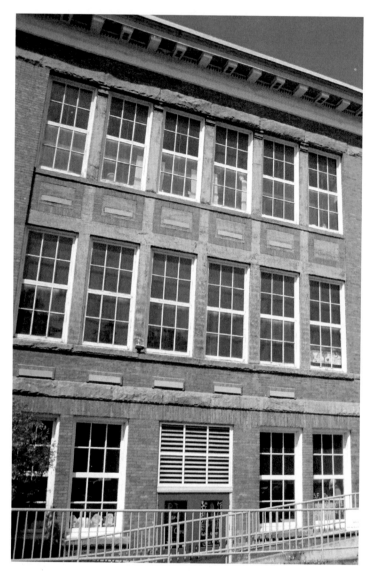

The 1916 wings at BF Day School were added during the peak of the open air school movement. They feature large center pivot windows that swing out, maximizing natural ventilation.

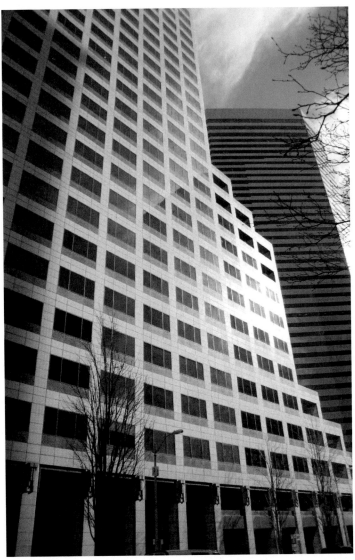

In many modern buildings, HVAC systems are used instead of windows to provide ventilation. These mechanical systems can help to create a comfortable indoor environment, but they do not provide much fresh air. This is a problem!

What is so special about fresh air?

Fresh air contains a *balance of positive and negative air ions*. Ions are charged microscopic particles (atoms) in the air. They are created in the natural environment when molecules are broken apart by sunlight and radiation, and by friction between air and water. Positive ions are formed by the loss of electrons, while negative ions are formed by the gain of electrons.

The numbers of positive and negative ions in the air are affected by natural and artificial influences in the environment. Dry weather, air pollution, air conditioning and electronic equipment increase the numbers of positive ions. Dispersion of water, such as through evaporation, waves, rain and waterfalls, increases the number of negative ions.

The positive benefits of negative ions

Negative ions, it turns out, are really *great* for our health. An abundance of negative ions increases the flow of oxygen to the brain, which in turn increases alertness and provides more mental energy. Negative ions also have a positive effect in reversing SAD and depression symptoms. In fact, studies at Columbia University have shown that exposure to large amounts of negative ions is *as effective as light therapy* for reversing depression.

When should we seek out negative ions?

When there is a long period of dry weather, positive ions increase and negative ions decrease. The same situation occurs indoors wherever HVAC and electronic equipment are used, and inside closed moving vehicles powered by combustion engines. If people spend hours in these environments, they may find themselves feeling tense, lethargic and depressed. This is because the reduction in negative ions increases airborne pollution, which triggers a response in the body.

Since most people are working indoors in air conditioned environments, it would make sense to deliberately seek out lots of negative ions to counteract the effects of these environments.

Spending hours in environments that are deficient in negative ions can leave people feeling tense, lethargic and *depressed*.

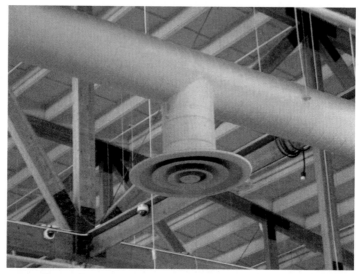

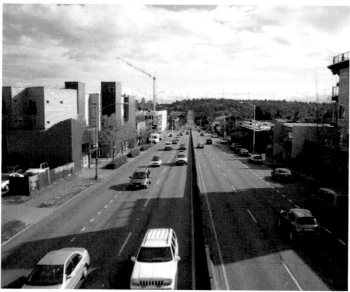

Air conditioned environments and closed moving vehicles (cars, buses, trains and airplanes) are likely to be deficient in negative ions, which can contribute to making people depressed.

Rain might be our best tool against SAD

Having learned that negative ions are plentiful near waterfalls, I wanted to know how *rain*, which *falls* so much here, would measure up. This inspired me to do some research on my own.

I recalled how especially invigorating it was to ride my bike in a heavy rain, so I decided to buy an air ion meter and measure negative ions under the same conditions. In measuring along the Burke-Gilman Trail in a heavy rainstorm, my meter registered the highest numbers of negative ions wherever rain splashed in puddles along the trail. I now understood why the harder it rained, the more invigorated I felt: more friction between air and water = more negative ions.

Could it be that all we need to do is get out in the rain and splash around in puddles?

Exposure to large amounts of negative ions has been found to be as effective as light therapy for reversing depression. Could the rain be Seattle's best tool against SAD?

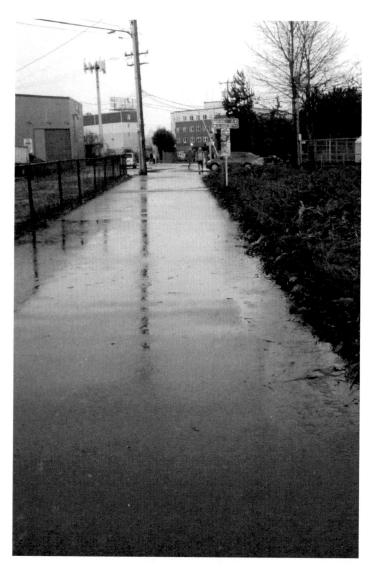

Although I expected to find lots of negative ions in a heavy rain, I was surprised at how much more abundant they were wherever rain splashed in puddles along the trail. Maybe splashing in puddles is exactly what we should be doing in the rain.

Forests and beaches offer negative ions

As part of my research, I took my air ion meter with me on a hike up Tiger Mountain. In measuring at a few locations along the way, I found that there were very high readings by a brook that tumbled over logs on its way down the hill. I expanded my research to some locations on the Olympic Peninsula. In the Hoh Rain Forest, I measured significant amounts of negative ions along the trail, and especially high numbers near waterfalls and runoff. At Kalaloch Beach, there were higher numbers whenever water spray drifted my way. It makes sense that kids are drawn to play in the surf!

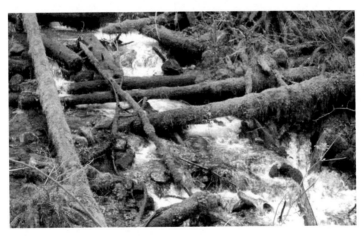

Hiking in the forest, it was not surprising to find that the highest numbers of negative ions were near a brook that tumbled its way over logs and rocks.

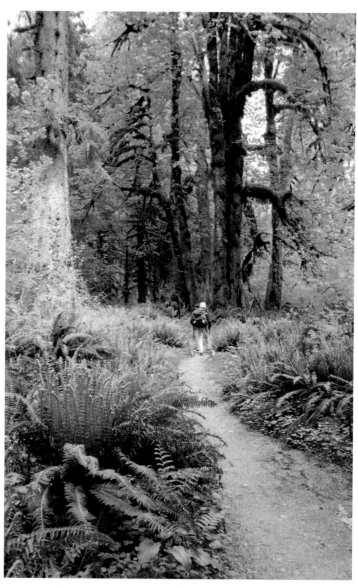

In the Hoh Rain Forest, I measured higher numbers of negative ions than in the woods on Tiger Mountain. Our native rain forest is a great place to go for lots of negative ions.

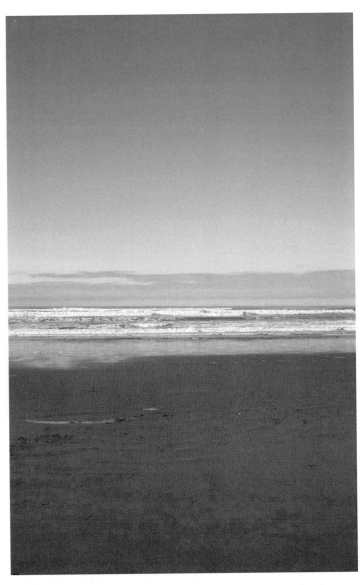

At Kalaloch Beach, the highest amounts registered whenever water spray drifted toward me. It is not surprising that kids like to play in the surf!

Seek negative ions outdoors - winter

If we are constantly exposed to air conditioned environments, we should find ways to counteract the negative health effects of these environments. In the wintertime, it would probably help to spend as much time outside as possible, *especially when it is raining.*

Layering clothes, such as adding lightweight nylon hiking pants over stockings or work pants, provides insulation and makes it more comfor table to walk in the wind and rain. If we can solve the comfort problem, we are more likely to spend time outside in the rain.

Exercising outdoors is not only a great way to get more negative ions, according to numerous studies, it helps to reduce depressive symptoms. Walking at least part of the way to and from work would help to ensure some exposure to fresh air (and thus more negative ions).

There are other ways to get fresh air on the way to the bus stop and to have fun getting there. My friend Eric uses a push scooter part of the way and always seems to be full of positive energy!

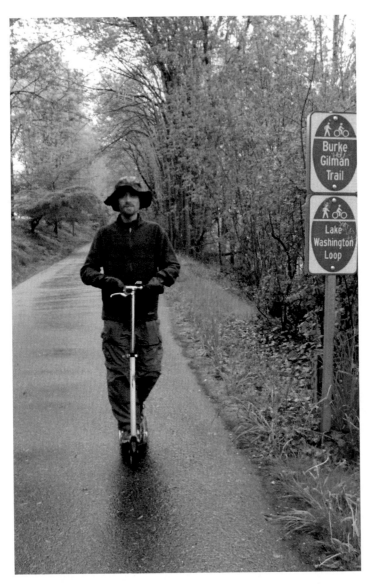

My friend Eric uses a push scooter to get himself to the bus stop on weekday mornings. This way, he is able to get lots of negative ions (and positive energy!) before starting work for the day.

Seek negative ions outdoors - summer

There are typically few rainy days in Seattle during late July, August and September. A long dry spell reduces the quantity of negative ions in the air. At these times, just going outside may not provide much relief from an air conditioned workplace. Where to find negative ions?

Since negative ions are found in abundance near waterfalls, I decided to take some measurements near the water fountain at Sculpture Park, on the Seattle waterfront. I took the measurements during a dry period in summer - next to the fountain, and half a block from it. The results indicated exponentially greater numbers of negative ions next to the fountain than half a block from it. During the dry months, people who work in air conditioned environments could be energized by lunching near a vigorous water fountain.

In addition to fountains, there are some powerful waterfalls located in parks and building plazas around downtown Seattle. My favorite waterfalls are in Waterfall Garden Park and Westlake Park.

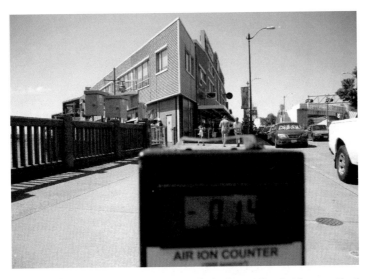

*During a hot dry spell, half a block from the Sculpture Park fountain, my meter measured **140 negative ions/cc**.*

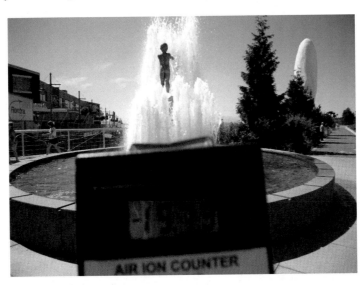

*Six feet from the Sculpture Park fountain, my meter measured a high of **15,130 negative ions/cc**, an exponential increase.*

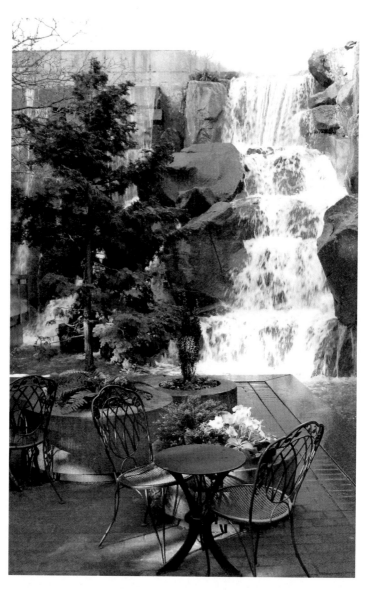

Prolonged dry periods in the summer reduce negative ions outdoors. The Waterfall Garden Park in Pioneer Square offers a refreshing location for a break or lunch hour.

126

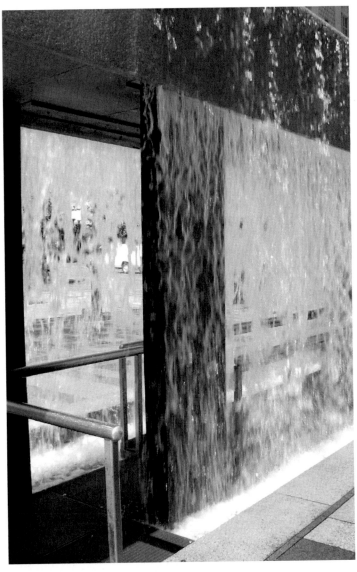

The water feature at Westlake Park includes a place to walk between cascading curtains of water. This would be a great place to get lots of negative ions!

Add negative ions indoors

At work, it should help to open a window (if that is possible) each day to bring in fresh air. A desktop fountain may help to improve the air quality within close range, such as at a workstation. There are also electronic air ionizers, but it is advisable to research their efficacy.

Adding a Himalayan salt lamp to one's work space is a positive way to increase exposure to negative ions, at least within close range. Salt therapy was used historically to treat tuberculosis and asthma after it was observed in the 1800s that salt miners did not suffer from the respiratory problems that plagued workers in other types of mines. Salt therapy is currently making a comeback as a natural therapy, with at least one treatment center opened near Seattle. A bath in Epsom salts would be a way to try out salt therapy at home.

Our homes have a built-in ionizer: a shower. Taking even just a brief shower can provide exposure to lots of negative ions. It could be just what is needed to restore balance after spending all day in an environment that lacks fresh air.

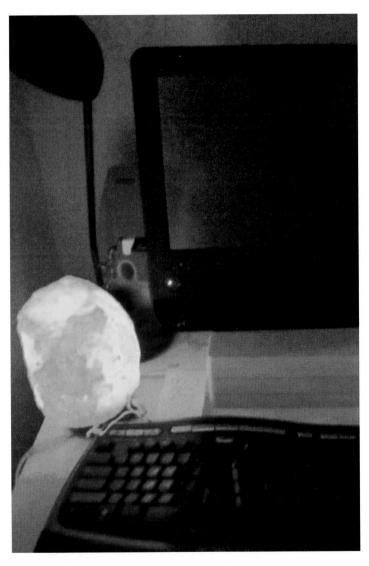

Himalayan salt lamps can increase negative ions within close range. The benefits of salt therapy were discovered in the 1800s, when it was observed that miners in salt mines did not suffer from respiratory ailments like workers in other types of mines.

Spending hours in air conditioned environments or closed moving vehicles exposes us to air that is missing the normal balance of ions found in fresh air. This change to the air can contribute to depression, lethargy and low energy.

We can improve our moods and energy levels by spending more time outside in the fresh air (especially in the rain), and in environments that offer abundant negative ions, such as near waterfalls, fountains, beaches and in the forest. Increasing negative ions indoors may also help. If we can become aware of how the air in our indoor environments may be affecting our moods and energy levels, we can take deliberate action to feel better.

The next chapter brings us to yet another helpful therapy for depression, one that has been used for centuries in other cultures to benefit people's health, including their moods: color therapy.

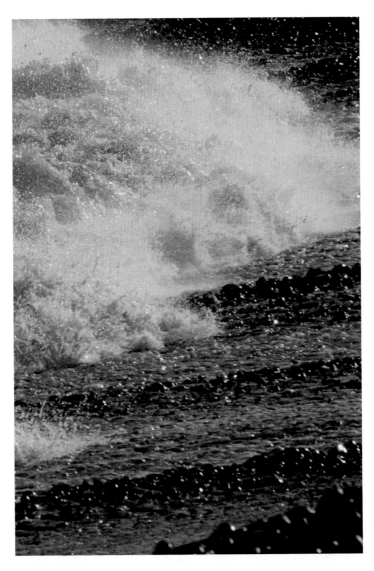

Lots of negative ions can be found at beaches with crashing surf, such as in Ballard, at Myrtle Edwards Park, and in West Seattle.

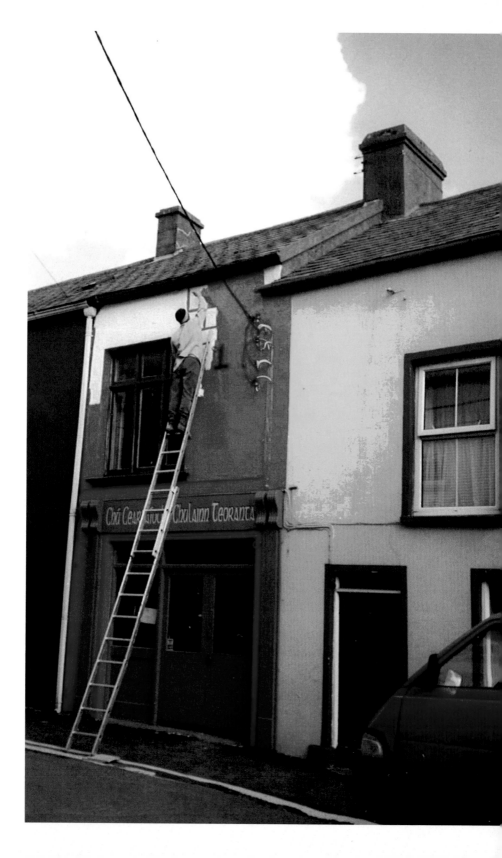

Chapter Five

Get Some Color!

Seattle - zero color in winter

In winter, Seattle suffers not only a deficit of daylight but also color. When the last of the seasonal flower displays have been removed, the predominant color left is grey: grey sky, grey buildings, and lots of grey pavement. The lack of color can make for a depressing urban environment, especially on dark days. On the occasional days when the sky turns blue overhead, people seem to go nearly crazy with relief!

During long overcast periods, people seem to respond enthusiastically to vivid colors, such as in flower bouquets, or even the bright pink of my Doc Marten rain boots. It is as if people are starved for color here in the winter, which might be the case.

Color is the most sacred element in all visual things.
~John Ruskin, 19th-century writer

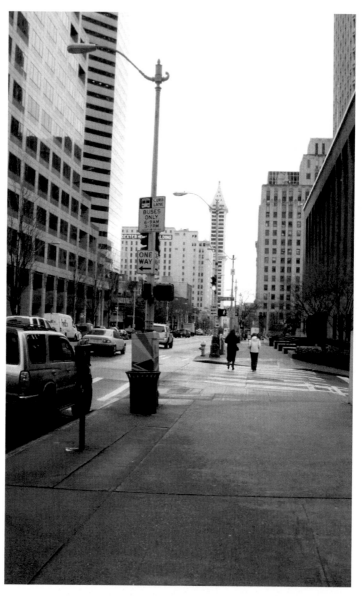

In winter, being surrounded by drab materials under a grey sky whenever we walk outside can be a very depressing experience!

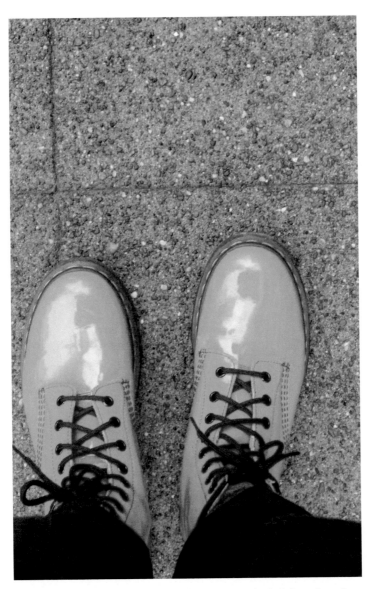

On gloomy days, people often exclaim over the bright color of my Doc Marten rain boots. It is as if people are starved for color here in the winter, which might be the case.

137

Color therapy was used as medicine

Color therapy (also known as chromotherapy) was used in ancient civilizations throughout the world to treat various illnesses, because it was believed that colors had healing powers. For example, in Egypt, special color rooms were used, and in Greece, the windows were covered with dyed cloths. Although color therapy continued to be practiced within Eastern medicine, it was viewed with suspicion (mostly as a pagan practice) in the Christian world and did not become part of Western medicine.

There was a re-emergence of interest in color therapy in the United States during the 19th century. Between 1861 and 1876, General A.J. Pleasonton experimented with the color blue and the health of plants, animals and humans. He found that alternating blue glass with transparent glass enhanced the growth of grape vines in a greenhouse, and that the use of blue light also cured diseases in animals and humans.

General Pleasonton's theory was never adopted by mainstream scientists. However, he was credited with the beginning of chromotherapy.

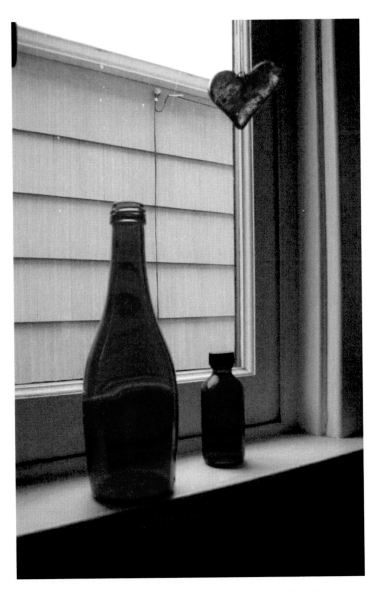

In the 19th century, adding strips of blue colored glass to greenhouses and structures was found to benefit the health of plants, animals and humans.

Pleasonton's research also led to a "blue glass craze", with people using blue glass to increase crop production.

Edwin D. Babbitt, also an American, pioneered the use of color to enhance human health, advocating for the replacement of drugs with natural remedies. The evidence that his color treatments were effective was great enough that the windows in many Victorian homes included colored glass to enhance the residents' health.

In the 1920s, American citizen scientist Dinshah P. Ghadiali determined that various parts of the body respond to particular colors. He promoted the use of color therapy to heal organs and body systems. His work and teaching helped expand interest and research on healing with color.

Although color therapy is not currently a mainstream treatment for depression, it appears to hold some promise. Studies began to focus on its potential in the 1990s, specifically on how color affects people's moods. A study from Vrije Universiteit in Amsterdam reported that adults felt happier around the colors yellow and green. Recent studies at the University of Freiburg showed that depressed people have a harder

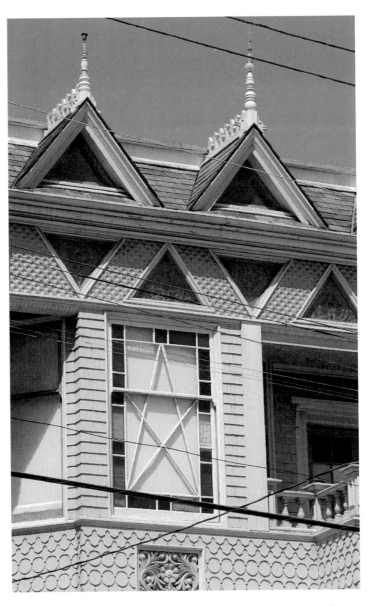

Colored glass was installed in the windows of Victorian homes because it was thought to enhance health.

time perceiving color, because the sensitivity of their retinas is decreased. The researchers suggested that color perception could be used as a new diagnostic tool and that color could be used to treat depression.

While the studies on the efficacy of using color therapy for depression are still ongoing, it seems to me that it can't hurt to experiment with it. Since Seattle has such a drab environment in the winter, any stimulation from color should help to cheer people up during the grey days.

Classic color therapy has usually meant sitting in colored light, such as using a colored gel in front of the sun or an artificial light. However, there may be other more practical and interesting ways to add color in order to stimulate energy and well-being. Visiting colorful places and adding more color to our wardrobes could help to increase our daily dose of color in the winter!

The nature of colour should change - no longer just a thin layer of change, but something that genuinely alters perception.

~Rem Koolhaas, Architect, Seattle Central Library

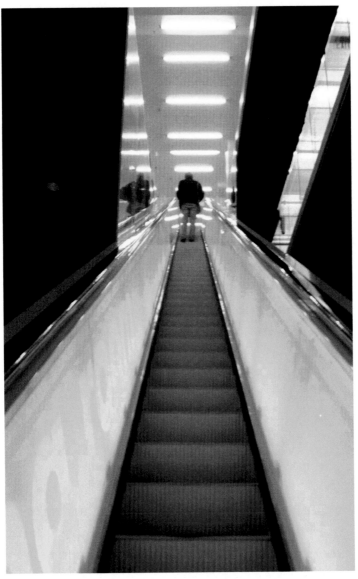

Neon green brightens the escalators and elevators at the downtown branch of the Seattle Public Library, providng a charge of color as people transit through the library's levels.

Spend time in a colorful environment

Spending time in colorful places can provide an uplifting experience in the winter. Walking through Pike Place Market, produce stands and flower stalls offer bright displays at eye level, where color is most needed. A visit to Volunteer Park Conservatory, with its rooms of lush green plants and bright flowers, could be just what is needed to boost one's mood on a dark day.

Other public places that offer lots of stimulating colors indoors include the downtown branch of the Seattle Public Library and the Seattle Art Museum.

Uplifting and stimulating colors can be added to our indoor environments by bringing in fresh floral arrangements. Bright flowers can also enhance the experience of sitting in front of a light box, providing a positive focus.

Painting warmer or brighter colors can help generate energy in dark or drab spaces. In my experience, transforming a dark living room by adding a warm orange color helped to make it a more cheerful space in the evenings and dark months.

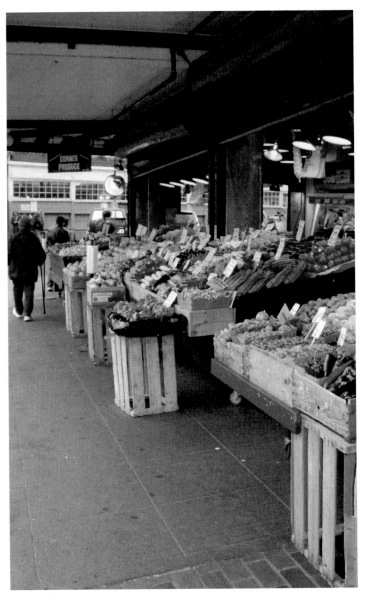

*A walk through Pike Place Market, full of colorful displays, is
sure to enhance a lunchtime walk on a grey day in winter.*

145

Wearing color brightens our moods

According to Catherine Cumming, an interior decorator and the author of *Color Healing Home*, people living in cities are more likely to wear black. "Black is absorbent and so can be draining and negative in its effect," she says. For people who feel depressed or lethargic, she suggests wearing uplifting and energizing colors such as orange and yellow.

Louise Hay, internationally renowned natural healer and author, says that wearing black "has a tendency to confine and repress the spirit" and suggests not wearing the color black for a month to see if we feel more cheerful.

According to modern color therapy, yellow and orange are helpful for alleviating depression. These colors are helpful to both the wearer and other people whose moods are brightened when they see them. Since color affects us individually, it probably makes sense to wear colors that appeal to us, that enliven us in the winter.

The next few pages show people who have dared to ditch the drab and wear colors instead.

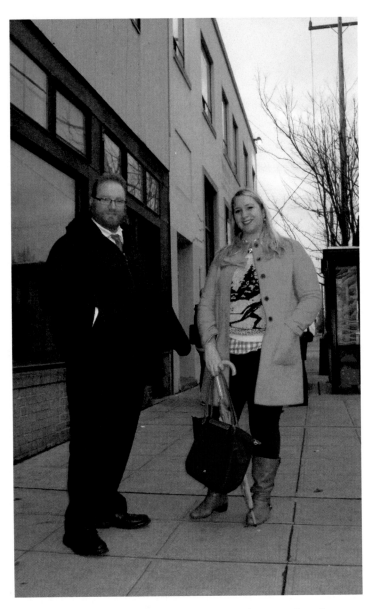

This woman's striking pink coat stands out in the grey environment and provides a dose of stimulating color!

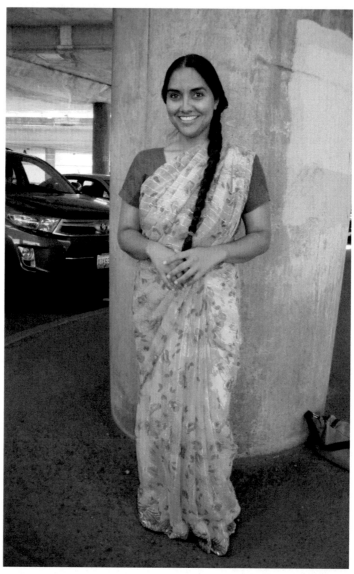

Although shooting this photo in summer required posing my friend in a parking area underneath the freeway, clearly her lovely yellow sari warms and cheers in any grey conditions!

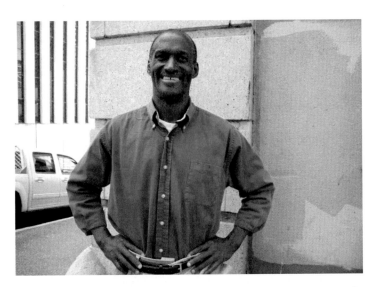

Fortunately, brighter colors have become more acceptable for men. It is good to see these colors against the grey!

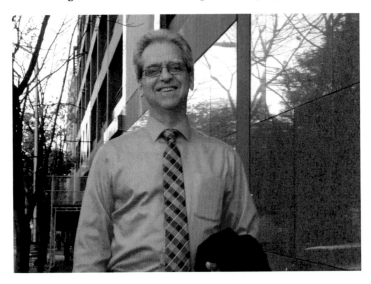

This gentleman's brightly colored shirt glows against the drab surroundings.

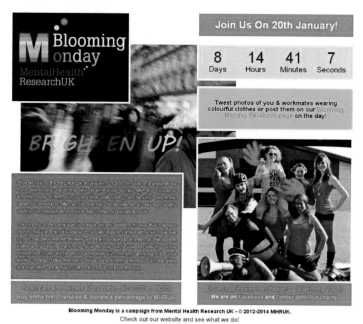

The Blooming Monday campaign in Britain promotes wearing colorful clothing to help fight the winter blues.

Could we use a "Blooming Monday"?

The issue of grey weather and SAD is being addressed in Britain through an innovative annual campaign, "Blooming Monday." On a Monday in January, people are encouraged to wear their brightest clothing. The idea is to lighten people's moods in the darkest part of the winter, when the holidays are past and spring is still far away. Perhaps a Blooming Monday campaign could be started in Seattle?

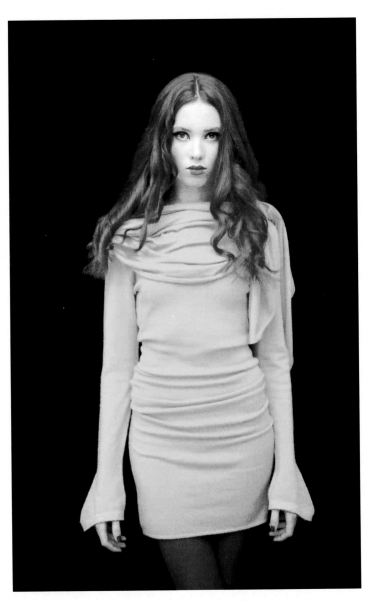

*This yellow dress by Rita Hraiz Colour Therapy Clothing (UK)
would certainly be appropriate to wear on Blooming Monday.*

Although the use of color therapy to treat depression is not yet well established, it seems that wearing bright colors and surrounding ourselves with them could only help us to feel better when long overcast periods (or hours inside an indoor environment) are making us feel *grey*.

The next chapter offers suggestions for changes to the built environment that would help people in Seattle to get enough light year round, and to provide a more stimulating environment during the long overcast periods here. There are many ways to beat Seattle's grey!

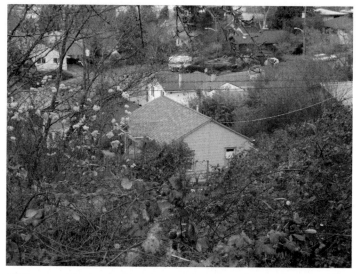

This orange house in Fremont adds a welcome boost to its drab surroundings in the winter. We need these sparks of color!

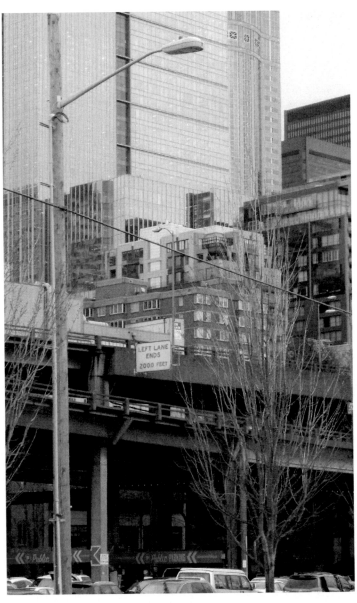

Why is the only bright color in this photo on a warning sign?
When there is no sun, we need more stimulating colors!

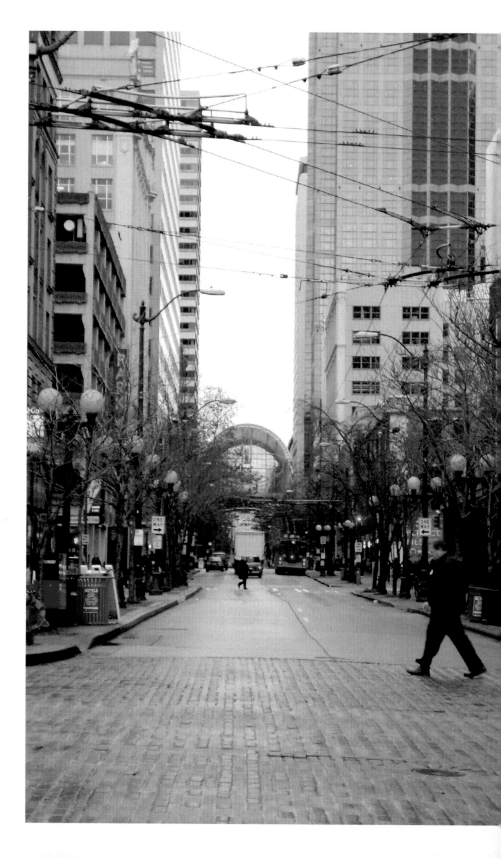

Chapter Six

How Could We Reduce SAD in Seattle?

Measure indoor light in the workplace

Insufficient bright light in the workplace contributes to the incidence of SAD in Seattle. Just like the housing styles found here, many building designs were copied from sunnier places around the United States, without consideration of the cloudiness and short winter days. People who work indoors are dependent on the quality of artificial light. Unless they go outside frequently or sit next to a bright window, most people get nearly all of their light during the day from overhead fixtures and desk lamps.

Workplaces with depressed employees are more likely to have sickness and absenteeism. For this reason, it would make sense to check light levels in work areas and to consider ways to increase the employees' access to bright light. Given the current standards in artificial lighting, most workplaces probably have illuminance consistently less than 500 lux except where work stations are located immediately adjacent to windows. This is much lower than the minimum 2500 lux necessary to reset our body clocks. Something needs to be done!

Expanding the use of light therapy: examples from Sweden

In Sweden, light therapy is used at businesses, nursing homes, hospitals, schools and even bus stops. Light therapy is accepted as *beneficial and necessary* for people's mental health if they do not have access to enough bright light, such as on short winter days.

In her book *A Life In Lux: Bright Insights About Wellness*, Swedish author Hippas Eriksson explains how light treatment helped to reduce use of sick leave and increased worker satisfaction and productivity, citing several examples where light treatment was incorporated successfully into work environments in Sweden. Some of these cases are described on the next pages. In one case, a

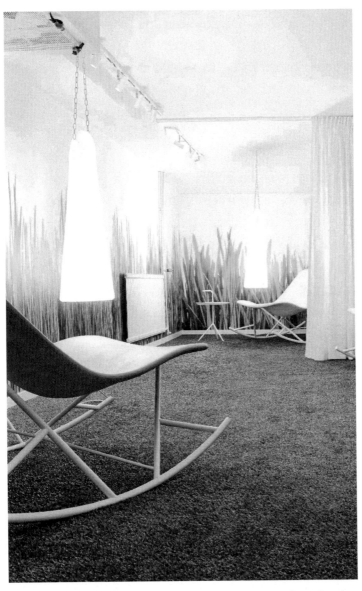

The use of light therapy has become mainstreamed in Sweden, such as incorporated into this relaxation room at Freys Hotel in Stockholm.

hospital added a light therapy room. The staff used the room as a lounge for relaxation and breaks. Some chose to read a book or just enjoy music played in the background. Employees reported that they felt more alert; others said that it gave them a harmonious feeling.

In another case, a business added a light therapy room for its employees. The room was ready in December, and they decided to form a test group to use it. The test group used the room for one hour a day over a two week period. It soon became obvious that even short periods per day yielded positive results. Too much time in the room caused disturbed sleep for some individuals. With the right balance of time, people who used the room experienced a better night's sleep and were happier and more active during the daytime.

In a third case, a nursing home changed an ordinary room into a simulated tropical paradise (see next page), including an artificial sandy beach with simulated sunlight and heat. Both staff and patients were able to use the room. Staff absenteeism was reduced by 25%. People who used the room reported that they

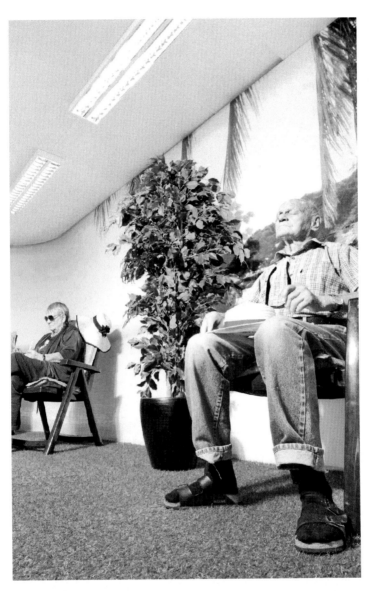

In this photograph by Swedish photographer Henrik Sellin, residents at a nursing home in Österåker, Sweden are shown receiving light therapy in a specially designated room.

felt healthier and more energetic. Clearly, light therapy is providing a benefit to these people.

Light rooms

Perhaps it is time to accept and incorporate light therapy as a necessary and healthy addition to workplaces in Seattle. It could help to add light rooms in workplaces, at least for use in the wintertime. Perhaps a section of a break room could be made into a light treatment area, outfitted with a few light boxes at a table. Standard therapeutic light boxes (10,000 lux) cost about $150-$300 each and require two fluorescent bulbs. These bulbs last a long time and are inexpensive to replace.

Light cafes

Light therapy could also be added to cafes. In Sweden, "light cafes" have opened to provide light therapy in the winter. One coffee shop in Seattle, Hotwire Coffee, has added light boxes. If light therapy were offered at more cafes, it would help people to add bright light daily at places they already frequent.

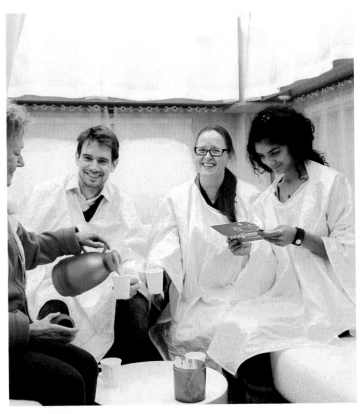

A mobile light cafe brings relief to Swedes in need of bright light therapy during short winter days.

Although this Swedish mobile cafe uses white fabric and robes to reflect the light, certainly light therapy can be less formal - it just requires a light box. Hotwire Coffee in West Seattle has added light boxes as an amenity for their customers. Hopefully other cafes in Seattle will consider adding light therapy, too!

Redirecting natural light

The benefits of the full-color spectrum of outdoor light cannot truly be duplicated with artificial lighting, therefore we ought to be maximizing the use of natural light wherever possible. Fortunately, new methods and lighting technologies are now making it possible to extend the reach of natural light inside buildings and into outdoor areas shaded by tall buildings.

One method, currently being tested in Scandinavia, uses solar collectors and fiber optic cables to transfer natural light. The technology transports the light but not its heat or ultraviolet radiation. An example of the lighting effect is shown on the next page. Another approach, using mirrors and metal ductwork, is under development in Canada and the United States.

Redirecting sunlight also offers a solution for increasing illumination in alleys and streets within dense urban areas. In Egypt, researchers in Cairo are developing a method that uses corrugated plastic panels angled on top of buildings to reflect light into streets below.

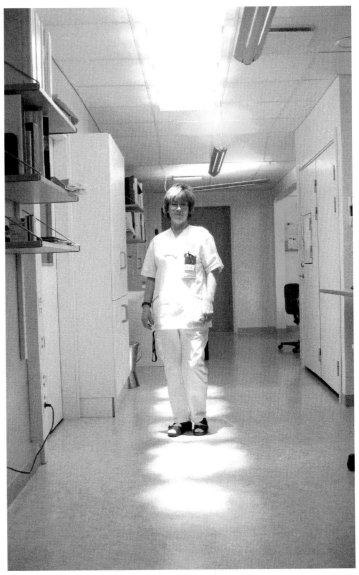

This photo shows an example of how natural light can be redirected inside a building using solar collectors and fiber optic cables. The light is transferred without its heat or UV radiation.

In modeling their use, it was determined that the panels could potentially increase illumination in the streets by 400% during the winter.

Another way to add light to dark areas outdoors is through the use of *heliostats,* mirrors that track the sun and redirect it as needed. In 2005, the Battery Park City Authority in New York installed three 8' heliostats (shown below) to follow the sun and redirect the light into a shady courtyard. The lighting effect from the heliostats is shown on the next page.

Perhaps panels and heliostats could be used to illuminate parks and streets as taller buildings create more shade in Seattle?

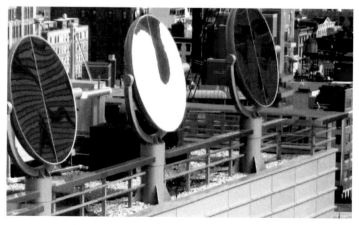

Heliostats installed on a building in New York City track the sun and redirect it into a nearby building's courtyard.

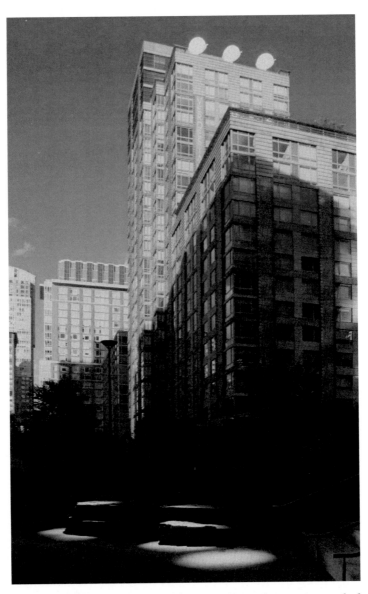

This photo shows how the heliostats redirect the sun into a dark courtyard. Might there be use for this technology in Seattle, as more tall buildings are added?

167

Atria add daylit space

In the early 1800s, atria were constructed in industrialized Britain as places for relaxation and gathering. Although the importance of daylight to health was not yet fully understood, people were drawn to these pleasant spaces.

In his 1816 book, *Fragments on the Theory and Practice of Landscape Gardening*, British landscape designer Humphry Repton promoted private atria as a way to improve the enjoyment of one's home through adding more natural light. Illustrations from his book, on the next page, show that adding more glass on both the sides and overhead (toplighting) improves the illumination of the space. They also appear to show the occupants smiling and relaxing in the atrium's natural daylight.

By the 1850s, private and public atria were common in Britain and Europe, and had spread to the United States as well. The first World's Fair in the United States was held in 1853 at the Crystal Palace in New York, a giant atrium built specifically for the Fair. Atria were also constructed to illuminate public places such as train stations and botanical gardens.

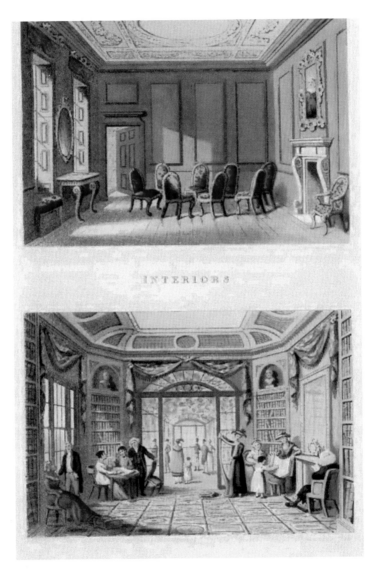

In his 1816 book, Fragments on the Theory and Practice of Landscape Gardening, British landscape designer Humphry Repton advocated the addition of more windows and toplighting (overhead glazing) to improve the light in an indoor space.

169

In some cases, public atria were built as a respite from air pollution in industrial areas. For example, the People's Palace and Winter Gardens (photo below) were built in the 1890s in East Glasgow, Scotland as a cultural center for residents when the city had become polluted and crowded. Today, the enclosed gardens provide a bright daylit community space for people to enjoy year round.

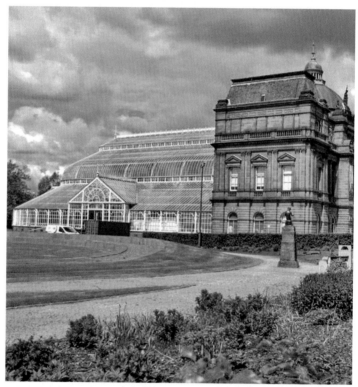

The People's Palace and Winter Gardens were built in the 1890s as a cultural center for residents in Glasgow, Scotland.

In Seattle, we need weatherproof public gathering spaces that provide us with the same amount and quality of light found outside. We need *greenhouses for people.*

The atria that are already incorporated into downtown Seattle buildings (listed in Chapter Three) provide access to daylight and include gathering space, but they typically include large overhead beams or walls that block significant amounts of light. For that reason, the illuminance inside them does not compare to the bright illuminance in greenhouses or outdoors.

The Volunteer Park Conservatory (shown on the next page) provides an ideal daylit weather protected space, but it was built for showcasing plants, not as a gathering space. It would help people to get more light if there were public atria designed similarly to the Conservatory, with minimized framing elements to allow in maximum daylight. They do not have to be designed as elaborate decorative structures such as the Conservatory or other early atria, however; they just need to provide us lots of natural light!

In Seattle, we need greenhouses for people!

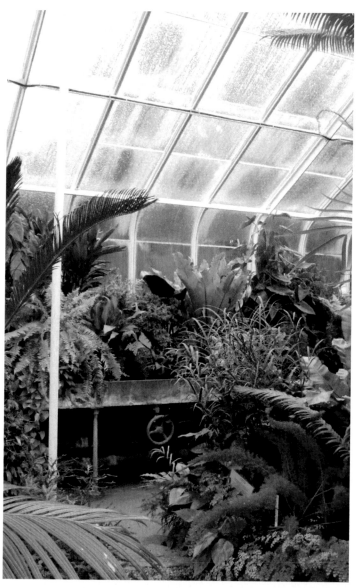

We need more bright daylit public spaces like the Volunteer Park Conservatory, but they should be built for gathering space, not just to showcase plants.

Exposed open spaces such as building plazas, parks and the Seattle waterfront could provide the benefits of daylight to the public year round if atria were added for weather protection.

The photo below shows a small freestanding atrium used as a park office and cafe in Iceland; I found these atria used commonly for private and public spaces there. Even a small atrium such as this one would invite people to go outside of their dark offices to get more daylight.

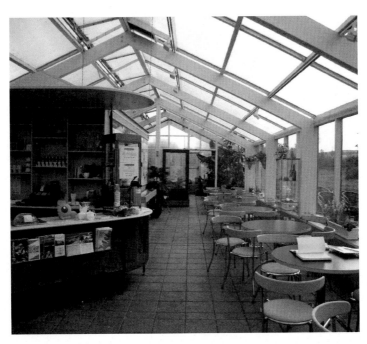

This small atrium in Iceland provides a pleasant daylit space. I think we could use these all over Seattle!

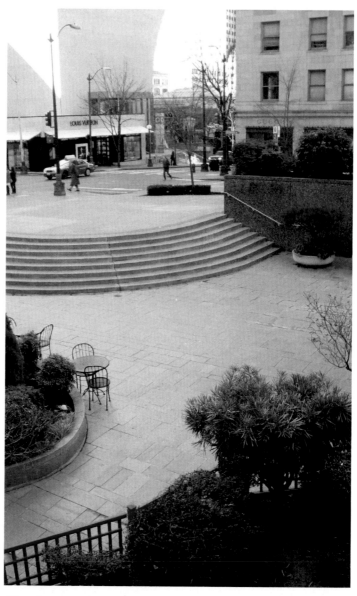

The plaza at 5th & University is an example of where an atrium could be added to provide a weatherproof daylit space.

174

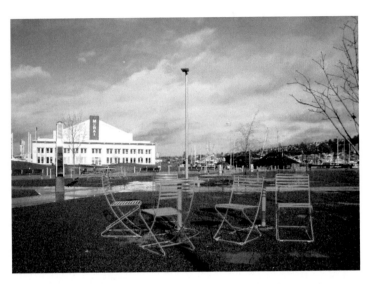

This public seating area at South Lake Union Park does not receive much use because it is exposed to the weather.

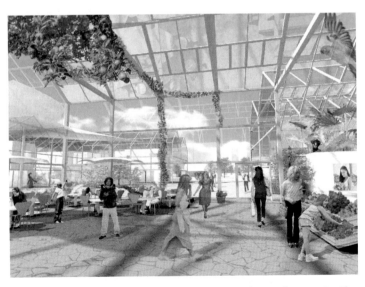

A public atrium could provide year round weather protection and daylit space for the seating. (Design by ASK Architects)

175

Daylighting buildings

Daylighting (illuminating buildings by natural light) can be incorporated into both new and existing buildings. This approach helps bring more natural light to people indoors, where they already spend most of their time. The description below and the photos on the next few pages explain how an existing building was retrofitted to help increase daylight. Perhaps these techniques could inspire changes to buildings in Seattle that would mitigate their dark design.

Eymondsson Bookstore in downtown Reykjavik includes daylighting features (designed by ASK Architects in Reykjavik) that were added some years after the building was constructed. An angled curtain wall was added to the front facade on both the second and third stories. A counter with seats was installed at the curtain wall on both floors, providing a view out to the street below. At the second floor, an atrium was added for a cafe, with a deck beyond it.

Visiting on grey days, I found that these spaces provided lots of natural light, and that people actively used them for reading and socializing.

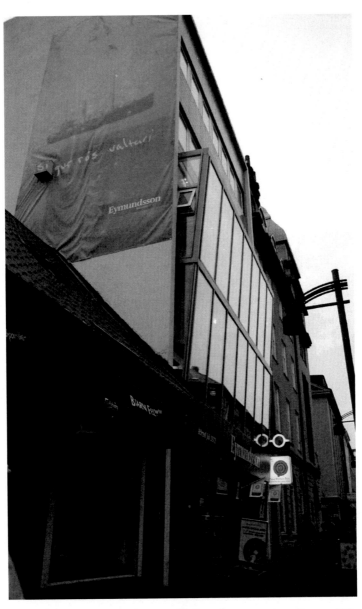

*An angled curtain wall was added to the upper two floors of the
Eymondsson Bookstore in Reykjavik.*

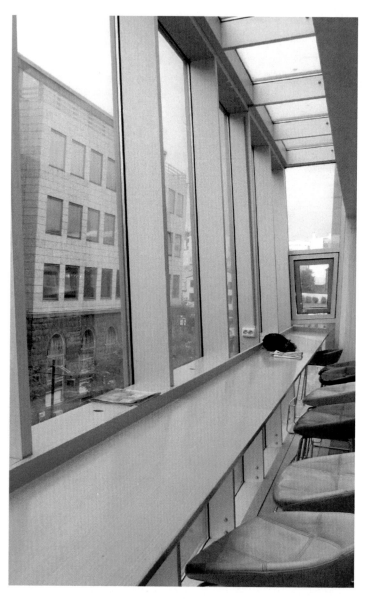

Counters and seats installed at the curtain wall on both levels provide a view of the street below.

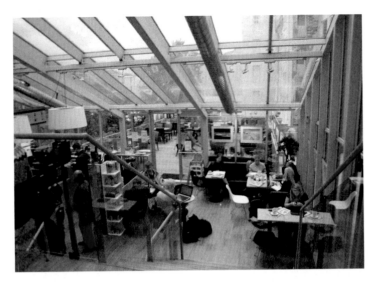

An atrium incorporated in the second floor of the Eymondsson Bookstore provides a bright and welcoming cafe space.

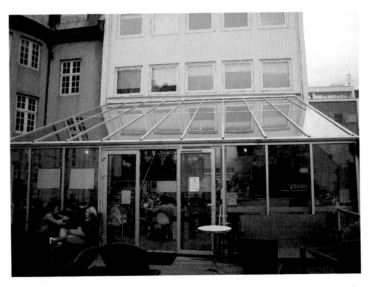

Beyond the atrium, a deck adds another opportunity for customers to gather in daylight, at least seasonally.

New daylit structures in Seattle

Some new structures have been built (or are currently proposed) in Seattle that are clearly being designed to respond to people's needs for natural light. This trend seems to signal that building science is at last committed to prioritizing the occupants' health. Several examples are cited below.

The new U.S. General Services Administration Federal Center South in SW Seattle, designed by ZGF Architects LLP, incorporates an atrium the length of the horseshoe-shaped building. The enormous skylight provides ample light for breaks from the darker workspaces in the building. Employers and restaurants are also starting to incorporate atria to provide naturally daylit spaces. For example, the new Amazon headquarters in Seattle, designed by NBBJ, will feature three domes that include workspace for employees. Also, Roberto's Venetian Restaurant in Pike Place Market includes a freestanding atrium designed by Atelier Drome Architecture. Photos and a rendering (computer graphic image) of these new daylit spaces appear on the next few pages.

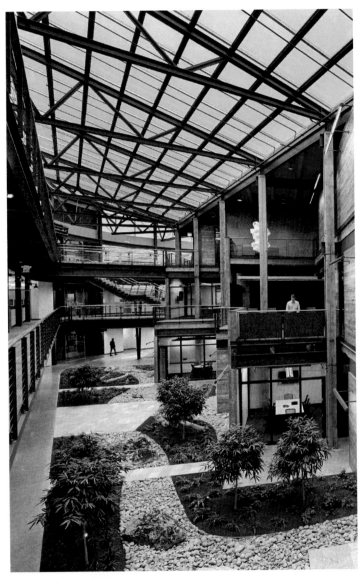

The US General Services Administration Federal Center South, designed by Zimmer Gunsul Frasca Architects LLP, features a skylight the length of the horseshoe-shaped building.

181

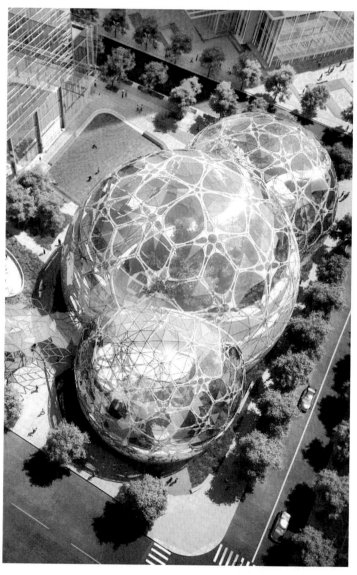

The new Amazon headquarters in downtown Seattle, designed by NBBJ, include transparent domes. This is excellent news for the employees, who will be able to work inside them.

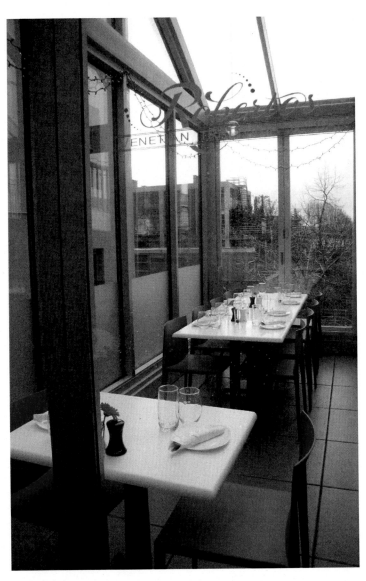

An atrium designed by Atelier Drome LLP provides a naturally daylit dining space at Roberto's Venetian Restaurant in Pike Place Market.

Adapting existing outdoor daylit spaces

It is encouraging to see the efforts being made to add more daylit spaces in Seattle. These improvements should help people who spend their workdays indoors have access to more natural light. Adapting outdoor spaces at existing buildings that already have toplighting would also add more opportunities.

For example, the primary entry to the Columbia Tower Plaza, shown on the next page, features a large skylight overhead. If a curtain wall were added, the space could be transformed into a weatherproofed daylit public seating area.

Another opportunity might be to add outdoor seating areas under transparent awnings. In Norway, cafe patrons are kept warm while sitting outdoors in the winter using portable heaters and blankets. Activating sidewalk space in Seattle during the winter would help to draw more people outdoors, increasing their exposure to natural light. Adding lots of daylit spaces would provide opportunities for people to get the light they need to thrive during Seattle's winters!

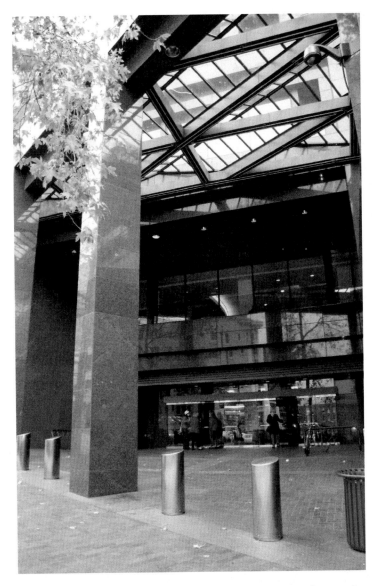

The entry to the Columbia Tower Plaza, exposed to the weather but covered by a skylight, could be made into a daylit public seating area if glass were added on the west side.

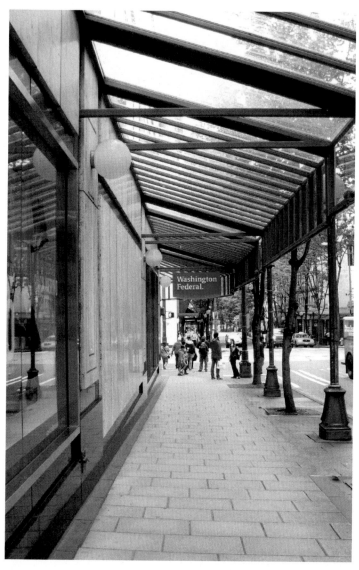

Transparent awnings such as this one at Fifth Avenue and Pine Street could provide excellent daylighting for outdoor seating areas. In Norway, cafe patrons outdoors are kept warm using portable heaters and blankets. Could we try this in Seattle?

Daylighting residences

Incorporating weatherproof daylit space in residences could be another way to mitigate light deficiency from an indoor lifestyle. The photos below and on the following pages show how balconies at residential buildings in France and Iceland have been mostly/fully enclosed in glass to enable their use year round. Perhaps adding glass to balconies would encourage people in Seattle to use them in the winter, for more light?

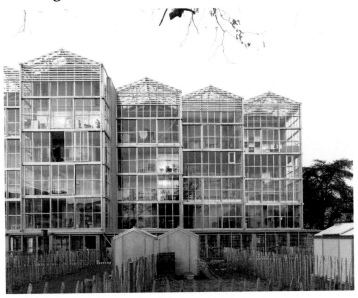

The BORÉAL® development in Nantes, France was designed by Tetrarc Architects to incorporate large daylit balconies on one side of the building.

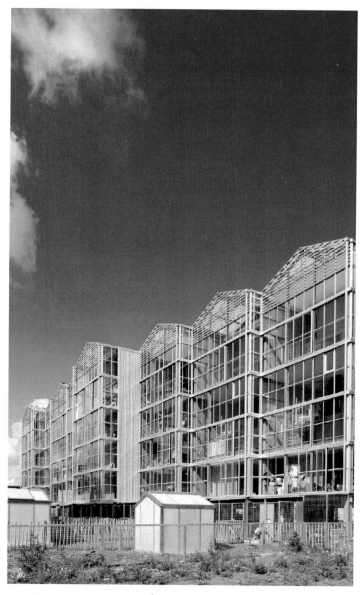

Another view of the BORÉAL® development. The balconies look out over garden plots, another healthy amenity for residents.

188

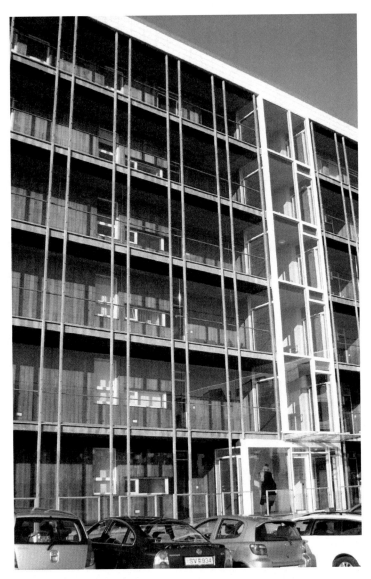

Shared balcony space at an apartment building in Reykjavik has been mostly enclosed with glass, providing weather protection while still allowing natural ventilation.

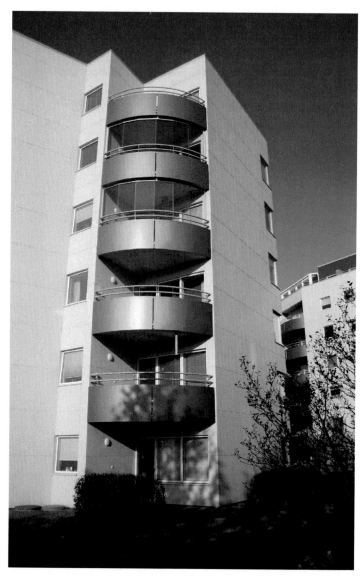

This multifamily building is one of several examples in Reykjavik where the residents can choose to have glazing added to their balconies for weather protection.

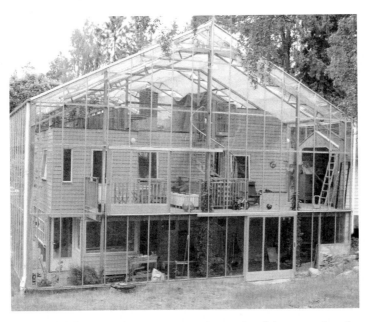

A greenhouse is built around a house in this example of a Naturhus (Nature House) in Ingaröstrand, Sweden.

In Sweden and Norway, enclosing a house within a greenhouse provides an innovative way to add more natural light and save energy for the homeowners. The home pictured above is an example of a "Naturhus" (Natural House), a design created in the 1970's by Swedish architect Bengt Warne.

The occupants are able to use their outdoor spaces and to grow fruit and vegetables most of the year. Because of the insulating glass, they also have significant electricity savings.

More color for Seattle

As mentioned earlier, the predominance of drab colored building materials in downtown Seattle contributes to a depressing pedestrian environment in the winter. Why is it that the only color you see in the winter is on warning signs, advertising, or taxis? I think more could be done to add bright, life-enhancing colors to the built environment. More color could draw us outside downtown!

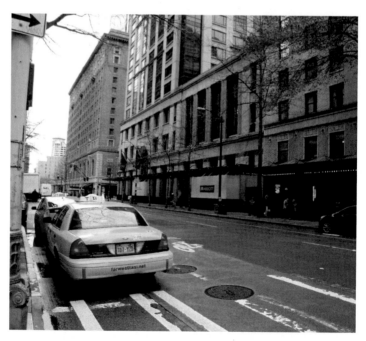

In the winter, sometimes taxis are the most colorful sight to be seen in the drab pedestrian environment.

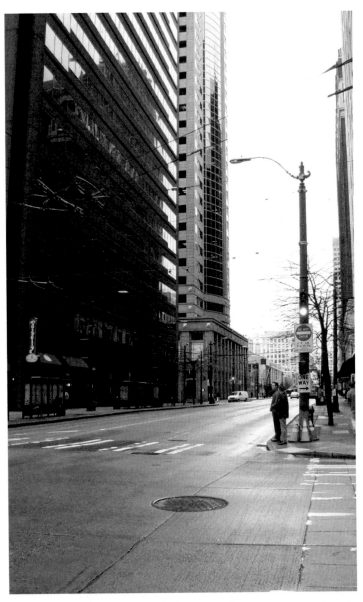

There should be ways to add more color at street level, besides signs, to enliven the experience of a pedestrian!

There is hope and stimulation in the addition of color. Perhaps Ireland can set an example for us? Ireland's marine climate is similar to Seattle's, with many grey days. But in contrast to the drab colors found here, buildings are repainted in bright colors as part of "Tidy Town" competitions that are held annually. The competitions were started in the 1950s to improve social conditions during an economic depression. Ireland is not alone in this approach. A former mayor in Albania, Edi Rama, used the addition of color on buildings to lift morale in the city. An unexpected positive outcome was a reduction in civil disorder.

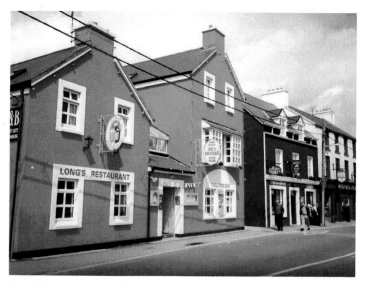

Brightly painted buildings in Dingle, Ireland liven up the streetscape on grey days.

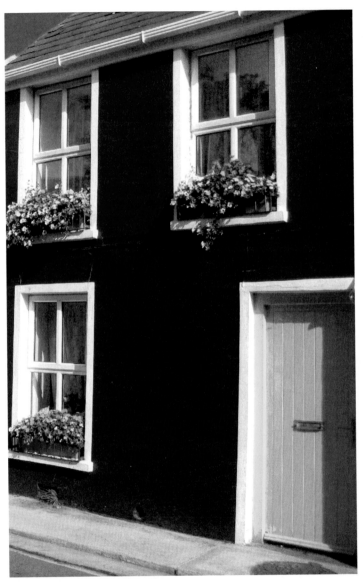

Canary yellow doors and flowers complement the intense color of this cobalt blue house in Dingle.

It is possible to find some exceptions, but mostly the chosen palette for colors on buildings in Seattle seems to be beige and grey, along with some other earth tones. Could we add more bright colors, such as yellow?

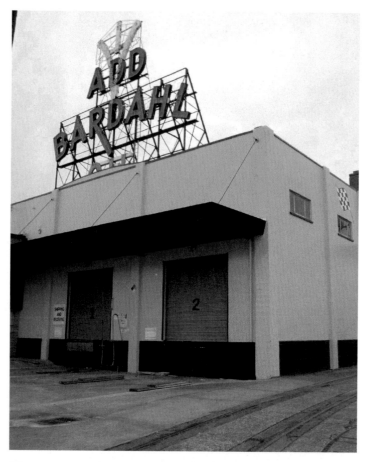

The canary yellow Bardahl Oil Building glows cheerfully against the gloomy skies over Ballard.

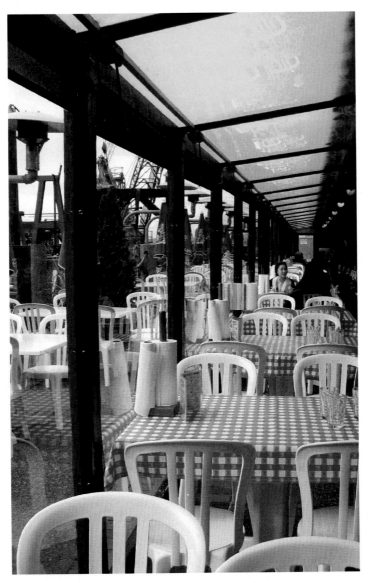

A yellow material attached to the skylight softens and colors the light over part of the dining area at the Crab Pot Restaurant on the Seattle waterfront.

Brightening business districts

Together with grey skies and asphalt, drab building materials reduce light and color in business districts. Perhaps this problem could be reversed through brightening the built environment by adding vibrant colors at street level. It should also help to draw more pedestrians.

Following the example of the Tidy Towns campaign in Ireland, buildings could be repainted in bright colors. If that is not practical, perhaps bright colors could be added other ways at street level, such as mounting brightly colored panels on walls or by adding colored lights under awnings, for use on grey days.

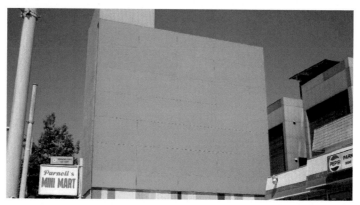

This bright orange wall in the Central District provides scintillating color at eye level. We need more bright colors!

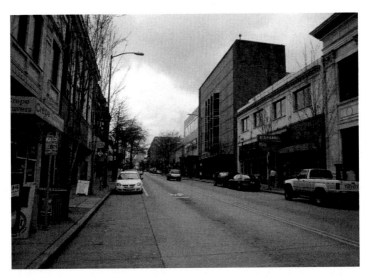

Drab colors. materials and pavement in the University District appear even more drab on grey days.

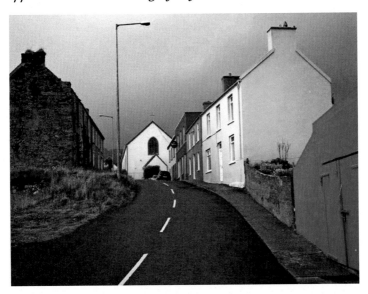

Could some buildings along the Ave be repainted in bright colors like towns in Ireland, to help counteract drabness on grey days?

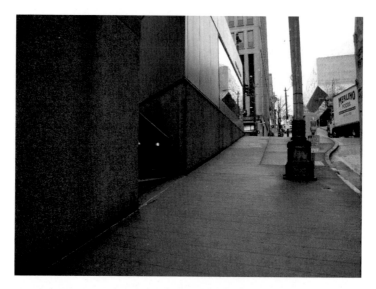

Drab colors can make it depressing to walk around Seattle.

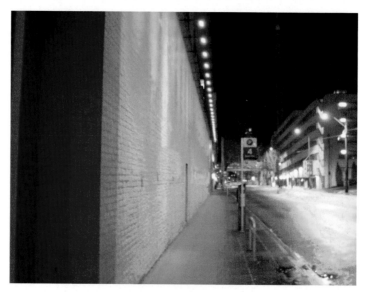

Installing brightly colored lights on walls or under awnings might help enliven sidewalks in the daytime on grey days.

More access to our open space

Each year, taller buildings are being added in neighborhood business districts and in downtown Seattle, encroaching on sunlight that used to reach pedestrian areas. It would seem crucial to replace these daylit areas to help people to get enough light daily.

According to the City of Seattle Department of Transportation, 27% of open space in Seattle is used for roads. Perhaps some streets could be closed to traffic, at least seasonally. Converting streets into pedestrian only areas has been shown to stimulate economic activity along them. In his book *Cities for People*, Danish architect Jan Gehl explains that creating these safe spaces *invites* people to walk and provides people watching opportunities.

"...in the industrialised world the ill-effects of sedentary indoor lifestyles are nearer the top of the public health agenda: obesity, heart disease, and depression, to name a few. And beneath all this runs an undercurrent of vitamin D deficiency. Medicine will not solve these problems. Prevention is required not treatment. Now it is the time for a built environment that puts health first."

~Richard Hobday, The Light Revolution

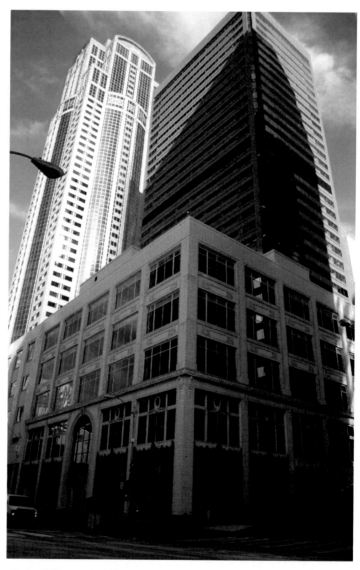

As buildings get taller in downtown Seattle and in neighborhood business disricts, more areas along the street become shaded. It would seem crucial to add space for people to get light outdoors. Closing some streets to traffic would help to reclaim open space.

202

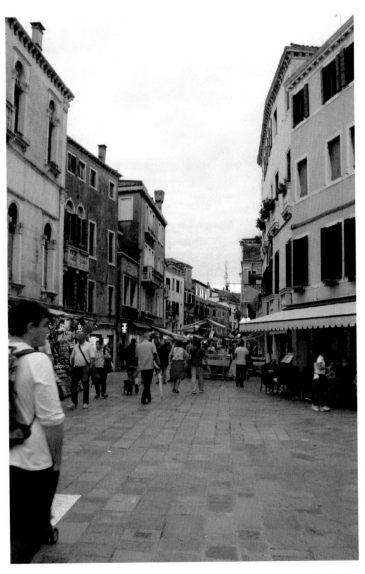

This photo shows a pedestrian-only shopping street in Venice, Italy. Creating pedestrian-only areas draws people outdoors to walk, and provides opportunities for people-watching. Since they are popular areas, they stimulate economic activity along the street.

Since most people are working indoors all day, a great deal are at risk for developing depression from light deficiency, especially in the winter. For that reason, changes should be made to the built environment to help increase people's access to outdoor, natural light. Daylighting buildings and adding public atria would go far to address the issue. In addition, new technologies that help to bring daylight inside buildings and illuminate shaded areas in the streets should be explored. Changes should also be made to improve Seattle's pedestrian areas so that they are enlivening rather than depressing in the winter, such as adding more color at street level, and by closing some streets to create safe places to walk and meet. These changes would help to draw people outside in the winter for light and fresh air, thus improving their mental health.

The final chapter explains how environmental influences such as low barometric pressure, air pollution and noise pollution can contribute to depression. Since these are all conditions that affect us in Seattle, more research should be undertaken locally to better understand their effects (and hopefully find solutions).

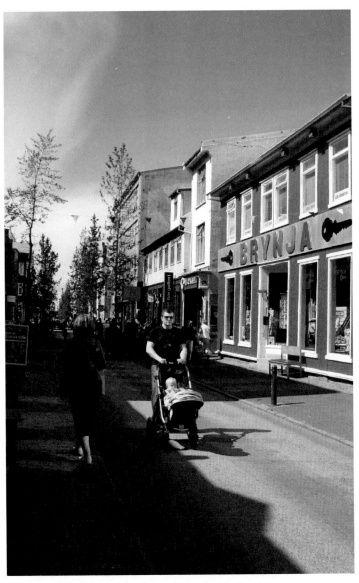

Adding pedestrian space in the street can provide more sunlight where sidewalks are shaded by buildings. This thriving shopping street in Reykjavik is closed to traffic seasonally.

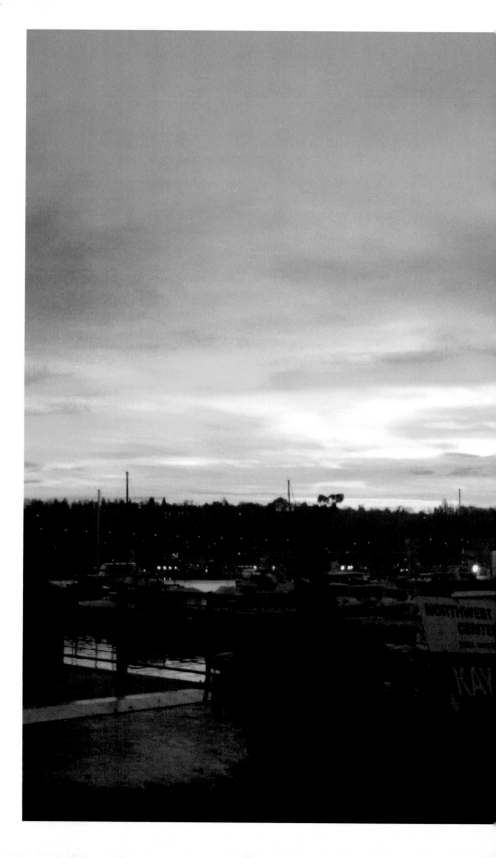

Chapter Seven

For Further Research...

Low barometric pressure

Barometric pressure is affected by weather and elevation. Low barometric pressure (1009 millibars and lower) is a known trigger for pain from arthritis and migraines. It is also associated with depression in some people, although it is not yet well understood why. Low barometric pressure exerts pressure on the sinuses, which can affect people's moods and energy levels.

Studies in Canada have found an association between low barometric pressure and suicide, and other studies have indicated that low barometric pressure aggravates depression-like behavior in rats. A 2008 Boeing study showed that when pilots were exposed to a drop in barometric pressure, they experienced lethargy. This was explained by the decrease in oxygen. Perhaps reduced oxygen would help explain the results in the other studies. Having learned that

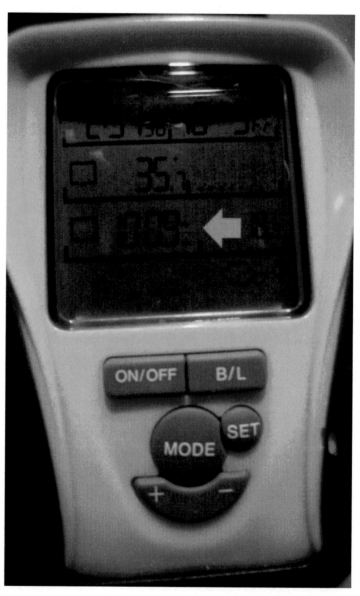

Low barometric pressure (1009 millibars or less) can bring on not only arthritis pain and migraines, but also depression.

low barometric pressure could be a contributing factor to depression, I decided to track barometric pressure at home for a year. I found that it averaged 1002-1008 millibars during the entire year. I next compared the barometric pressure at my workplace, located higher than my house, in a highrise building. I found that it was a few points lower than at home. This means that the places where I spend most of my time each day average low barometric pressure all year.

Since barometric pressure is also affected by elevation, I decided to compare it at sea level. It turns out that the barometric pressure at sea level is *eight* points higher than at my house. This means that when it is 1002 millibars (low) at my house, it is 1010 at sea level (normal). I was surprised that the location of my house at just 250 feet above sea level could make such a difference in barometric pressure.

Since barometric pressure is consistently higher at sea level, perhaps people who are affected by low barometric pressure should try living and working closer to sea level to see if it helps. In my personal experience, I have noticed feeling

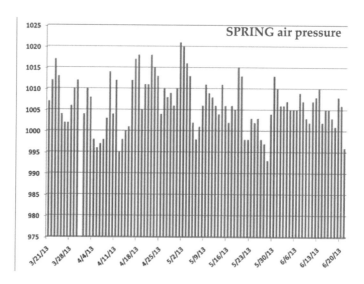

*Spring barometric pressure measurements at 249 feet above sea level in Seattle. Average: **1007 mb**.*

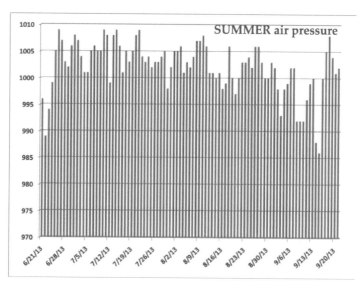

*Summer barometric pressure measurements at 249 feet above sea level in Seattle. Average: **1002 mb**.*

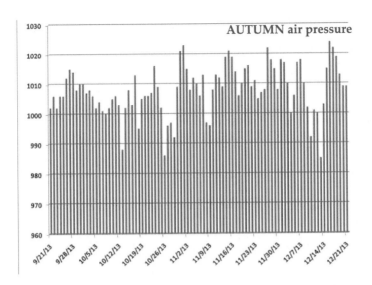

*Autumn barometric pressure measurements at 249 feet above sea level in Seattle. Average: **1008 mb**.*

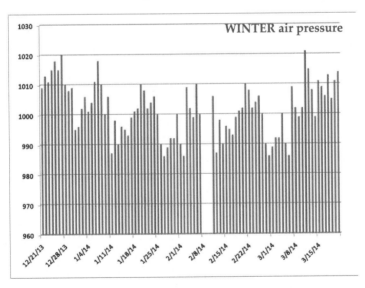

*Winter barometric pressure measurements at 249 feet above sea level in Seattle. Average: **1002 mb**.*

less energetic when the barometer drops below 1009 millibars. During low periods, I have also noticed that my sinuses become congested.

For people who are troubled by depression, tracking daily barometric pressure and recording changes to mood and energy level could help rule out the influence of low barometric pressure. Since elevation also affects barometric pressure, it would make sense to measure at home and work. The elevation of an individual address can be found by entering the address at http://www. heywhatsthat. com/profiler.html.

Air pollution

We have known for years that smog harms lungs and hearts, but new studies in Los Angeles and China have linked air pollution to depression also. One Chinese study indicated that even low levels of ambient pollution can impair one's ability to concentrate (a common symptom of depression). Although Seattle does not have chronic smog problems such as found in Los Angeles, we do have prolonged episodes

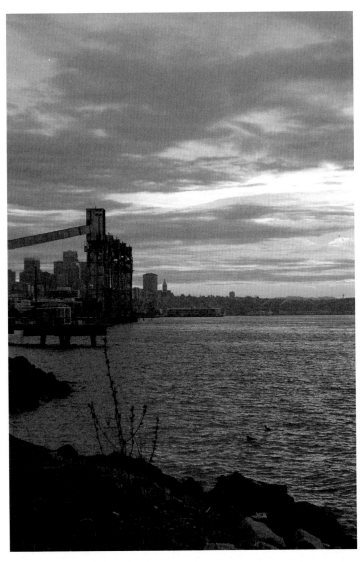

A moderate level of air pollution shows up as a tawny layer over the Seattle waterfront. Air pollution has been linked not only to lung and heart disease, but also to depression. Even low levels have been found to disrupt a person's ability to concentrate.

215

at times due to temperature inversions and stagnant air. Temperature inversions occur in Seattle because of the city's location between two mountain ranges. Inversions are layers of cold air above that trap rising warm air, causing smog to build downwards. They usually occur in late fall and winter, lasting a few days to a couple of weeks. Stagnant air can increase pollution levels anytime of year, because there isn't enough wind to blow the pollution away.

Even when the air quality is relatively good, the constant supply of vehicle exhaust and industrial emissions in Seattle means that we are always breathing air with some pollution in it.

To find out more about air pollution levels in my neighborhood and along my bike route to work, I bought an air quality monitor and started tracking the pollution myself. Sharing the data with staff at the Puget Sound Clean Air Agency has helped me to learn how to interpret the results of my measurements. Although my monitor is not as accurate as the scientific instruments installed by the Agency in several places around Seattle, the data helps their staff get a better picture of the levels of pollution at

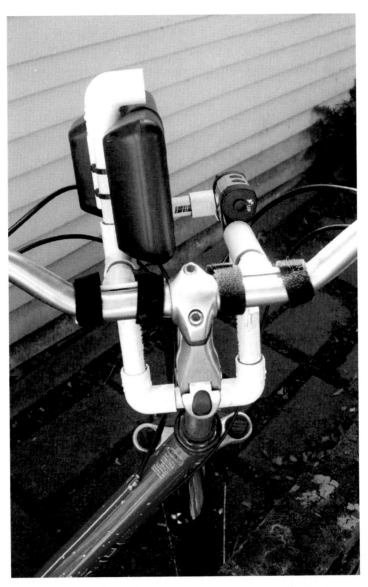

Tracking air pollution from the seat of my bike has helped me to understand more about the levels of air pollution found at ground level, where I am exposed to it while biking or walking.

ground level (where we are walking and biking!). As a result of my research, I am now more aware of when inversions are happening, what a moderate level of pollution looks like, and where higher levels of emissions are found. The most surprising thing I have learned is that fireworks can have a tremendous negative impact on the air quality in Seattle, for days.

For everyone's health (including mental health) we should be taking more steps to improve the air quality in Seattle. It would probably help if more individuals and groups such as schools tracked the air quality, because then it becomes more *relevant* to people's personal experiences. If people are made aware of how their own environments are affected by pollution, they are more likely to be motivated to help reduce it.

People who are sensitive to the effects of air pollution, especially those with asthma or heart disease, should check air quality daily. Information about current and predicted air quality in Seattle can be found on the Puget Sound Clean Air Agency's website at www. pscleanair.org. The website includes educational information.Since it has been established that

Since it has been established that even low levels of air pollution can affect people's mental health, it would make sense for local scientists to study how air pollution may be contributing to depression as a public health problem here.

Noise pollution

Researchers are finding that noise pollution also plays a role in depression. Although it does not cause depression directly, noise pollution can accelerate its development. Early studies focused on the effects of noise pollution on the development of children, but now there are numerous studies underway to better understand how noise affects adults.

Noise (unwanted sound) causes a fight or flight reaction in the human body, affecting the nervous, hormonal and vascular systems. The studies are finding that these effects of noise on the body increase the risk of depression and migraines. Even typical roadway noise levels have been found to elevate blood pressure. Noise at night disrupts people's sleep, which in turn makes it difficult to have a good mood the next day. Neighborhood noise, from other

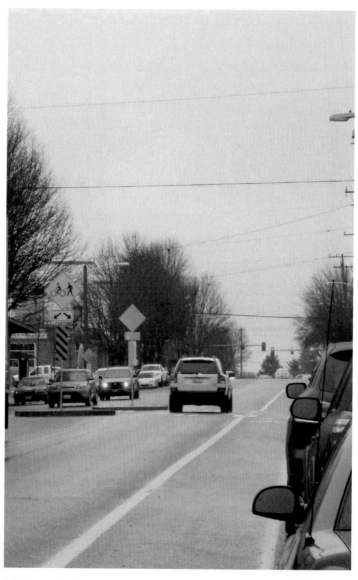

Noise pollution plays a role in depression because it elicits a fight or flight response in the body. Even typical road noise levels have been found to raise blood pressure.

properties or even within the home, can cause stress, since people spend so much time at home. Noise at work greatly matters, too: a recent study in Korea found that occupational noise was signif- icantly related to mental health, in particular, depression and suicidal ideation (thinking).

To help people in Seattle to thrive in our noisy urban environment, it would help to draw more attention to the issue through local studies on the subject of noise impacts to human health (and mental health). Perhaps noise regulations and designs could be modified to better protect human ears and reduce stress. One positive change would be to change emergency sirens to ones that use a lower frequency, an option that is still currently controversial but holds promise in reducing sound pollution.

As population density grows, protecting quiet in natural areas that provide relief from the noisy urban environment becomes especially crucial. One local campaign, One Square Inch of Silence, seeks to preserve quiet in the Olympic National Park: www.onesquareinch.org. Hopefully these efforts will expand to other natural areas.

Conclusion

Although Seattle's grey weather and short winter days can be challenging, they do not have to leave us suffering from SAD. Likely, the best solution for most people would be just to add more time outdoors each day, *especially* when it is raining (for negative ions). Adding more color to the pedestrian environment would help encourage people to go outside. Since not everyone can be coaxed outdoors, however, daylighting and atria should be added to provide more opportunities for people to get the benefits of natural, outdoor light. For everyone's health, it is time to start a *light* revolution in Seattle!

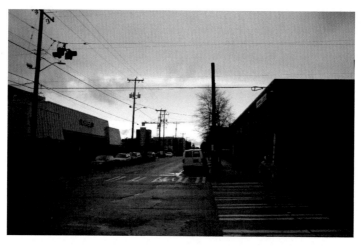

It is time to start a light revolution in Seattle!

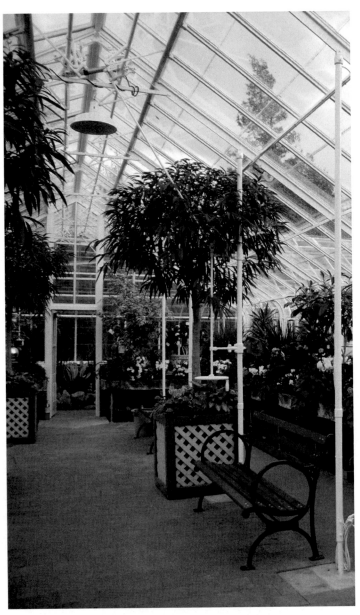

We need greenhouses for people!

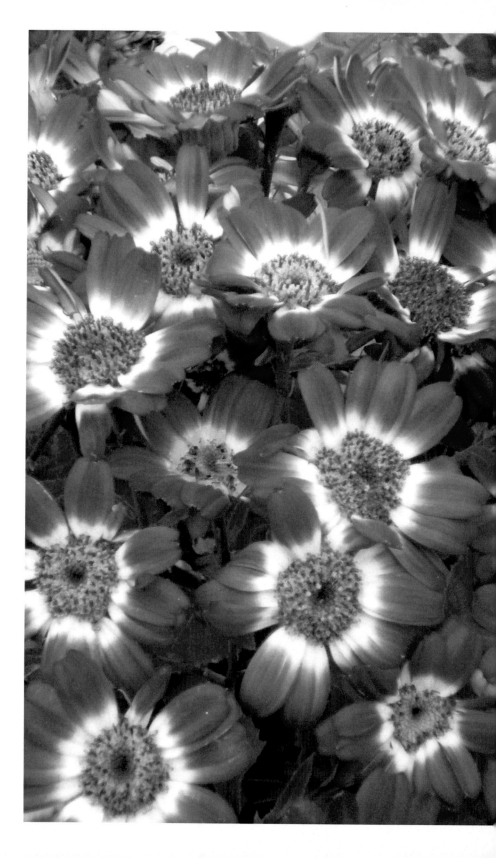

References

References

Azeemi, S., Raza, S. (2005). EA Critical Analysis of Chromotherapy and Its Scientific Evolution. *Evidence-Based Complementary and Alternative Medicine* 2(4): 481–488. doi: 10.1093/ecam/neh137 PMCID: PMC1297510

Bauer, J., Freyberg, R. (1946). Vitamin D intoxication with metastatic calcification. *The Journal of The American Medical Association*.130(17):1208-1215. doi:10.1001/jama.1946.02870-170014004

Becker, P. (2002). Firland Sanatorium, Seattle's municipal tuberculosis hospital, opens as Henry Sanatorium on May 2,1911. *HistoryLink.org.* Essay 390. Retrieved from http://www.historylink.org

Becker, P. (2002) Firland Sanatorium. *HistoryLink.org* Essay 3928. Retrieved from http://www.historylink.org

Beil, L. (2011, July 5). In Eyes, a Clock Calibrated by Wavelengths of Light. *New York Times.* Retrieved from http://www.nytimes.com

Blue light has a dark side. (2012, May). *Harvard Health Newsletter.* Retrieved from http://www.health.harvard.edu

Boubekri, M., Cheung, I., Reid, K., Wang, C., Zee, P. (2014). Impact of Windows and Daylight Exposure on Overall Health and Sleep Quality of Office Workers: A Case Control Pilot Study. *Journal of Clinical Sleep Medicine.* doi: 10.5664/jcsm.3780

Bubl, E., Kern, E., Ebert, D., Bach, M., Tebartz van Elst, L. (2010). Seeing gray when feeling blue? Depression can be measured in the eye of the diseased. *Biological Psychiatry.* 15; 68 (2): 205-8. doi: 10.1016/j.biopsych.2010.02.009.

Bullinger, M. (1989, June). Psychological effects of air pollution on healthy residents - A time-series approach. *Journal of Environmental Psychology.* 9:103-118

Campbell, M. (2005). What Tuberculosis did for Modernism: The Influence of a Curative Environment on Modernist Design and Architecture. *Medical History.*49(4): 463–488.

Carlowe, J. (2011, October 31). Coping with Seasonal Affective Disorder: A light café is the perfect place to lose those SAD 'winter blues.' *The Telegraph.* Retrieved from http:/www.telegraph.co.uk/

Cumming, C. (2000). *Colour Healing Home: Improve Your Well-Being and Your Home Using Color Therapy.* London: Mitchell Beazley.

Department of Planning & Development, City of Seattle. *Privately Owned Public Spaces.* Retrieved from http://seattle. gov

Dunn, A., Trivedi, M., Kampert, J., Clark, C., Chambliss,H. (2005, January). Exercise treatment for depression. *American Journal of Preventive Medicine.* 28: 1–8.

Eagles, J. (2003) Seasonal affective disorder. *British Journal of Psychiatry.* 182: 174-176. doi: 10.1192/bjp02.129.

Earthbeat - Architecture and Well-Being. (2010). *Radio Netherlands Worldwide.* Earth Beat reporter Marnie Chesterton interviews Dr. Norman Rosenthal. Retrieved from http:// www.rnw.nl/english

Eastman, R., Warren, S., Hahn, C. (2014). *Climatic Atlas of Clouds Over Land and Ocean* . Department of Atmospheric Sciences, University of Washington. Retrieved August 16, 2014 from http://www.atmos.washington.edu/CloudMap/

El-Mallakh, R., Nair, S., Piecznski, N., Schory, T. (2003). Barometric pressure, emergency psychiatric visits, and violent acts. *Canadian Journal of Psychiatry.* 48 (9): 624-7.

Eriksson, H., Brink., A. (2008). *A Life In Lux: Bright Insights About Wellness.* Stockholm: Hippas Productions.

Freund, D. (2012) *American Sunshine: Diseases of Darkness and the Quest for Natural Light.* Chicago, IL: University of Chicago Press.

Gehl, J. (2010) *Cities for People.* Washington, DC: Island Press

Glickman, G., Hanifin, J., Rollag, M., Wang, J., Cooper, H. Brainard, G. (2003). Inferior retinal light exposure is more effective than superior retinal exposure in suppressing melatonin in humans. *Journal of Biological Rhythms.* 18(1): 71-9.

Goines, L., Hagler, L. (2007). Noise Pollution: A Modern Plague. *Southern Medical Journal.* 100 (3): 287-294.

Haraszti, R. Purebl., G., Salavecz, G., Poole, L., Dockray, S., Steptoe, A. (2014) Morning-eveningness interferes with perceived health, physical activity, diet and stress levels in working women: a cross-sectional study. *Chronobiology International.* (7): 829-37. Doi: 10.3109/07420528. 2014.911188.

Harb, M., Paz Hidalgo, M., Martau,B. (2014). Lack of exposure to natural light in the workspace is associated with physiological, sleep and depressive symptoms. *Chronobiology International.* Vol. 0, No. 0: 1-8. doi:10.3109 /07420 528.2014.982757

Hay, Louise. (2010). *Colors & Numbers: Your Personal Guide to Positive Vibrations in Daily Life.* Carlsbad, CA: Hay House.

Hix, J. (1974). *The Glass House.* Cambridge, MA: MIT Press.

Hobday, R. (2007). *The Light Revolution: Health, Architecture and Sun.* Scotland: Findhorn Press.

Hobday, R., (1997). Sunlight therapy and solar architecture. *Medical History.* (4): 455-72.

Hobday, R, Dancer, S. (2013) Roles of sunlight and natural ventilation for controlling infection: historical and current perspectives. *Journal of Hospital Infection.* 84:271-282.

Innes, E., (2014, January 2) 10% of us go through winter without ever seeing sunlight during the week, increasing our risk of mental health problems. *UK Daily Mail.* Retrieved from http://www.dailymail.co.uk

Itoh, M., Funakubo, M., Sato, J. (2011). Lowering barometric pressure aggravates depression-like behavior in rats. *Behavioral Brain Research.* 218(1)190-3. doi: 0.1016/j.bbr. 2010.11.057.

Konnikova, M. (2013, December 10). Snoozers are, in fact, losers. *The New Yorker.* Retrieved from http://www. newyorker.com.

Light from self-luminous tablet computers can affect evening melatonin, delaying sleep. (2012, August 27). *Science Daily.* Retrieved from http://www.sciencedaily. com.

Lim, Y., Kim, H., Kim, J., Bae, S., Park, H., Hong, Y. (2012). Air Pollution and Symptoms of Depression in Elderly Adults. *Environmental Health Perspectives.*120(7): 1023–1028.

Macrae, F. (2014, April 2). A morning walk is key to losing a few pounds: Scientists say bright light helps regulate metabolism. *MailOnline.* Retrieved from http://www. dailymail.co.uk/

Manning, Harvey. (1986) *Walking the Beach to Bellingham.* Seattle: Madrona Publishers.

Mcfadden, E., Jones, M., Schoemaker, M., Ashworth, A. (2014) The Relationship Between Obesity and Exposure to Light at Night: Cross-Sectional Analyses of Over 100,000 Women in the Breakthrough Generations Study. *American Journal of Epidemiology.* 180 (3): 245-250. doi: 10.1093 /aje/kwu117

Mental Health Research UK (MHRUK). (n.d). *Blooming Monday Campaign.* Retrieved January 3, 2014 from http: //www.mhurk.org

Mizoguchi, H., Fukaya, K., Mori, R., Reed, C. (1934). Symptoms of Viosterol overdosage in human subjects. *The Journal of the American Medical Association.* 102:1745–1748.

Muhm, J. (2008) Effects of Mild Hypobaric Hypoxia on Oxygen Saturation During Sleep. *ClinicalTrials.Gov.* Retrieved from https://clinicaltrials.gov/

Negative Air Ionization. *Columbia Psychiatry, Columbia University Medical Center.* Retrieved November 14, 2014 from http://asp.cumc.columbia.edu/

Noise pollution: vehicles are the worst offenders. (2014, April 1). *Daily Tribune News.* Retrieved from http://dt.bh

Open Air School Movement. (n.d) *Encyclopedia of Children and Childhood in History and Society.* Retrieved May 5, 2014 from http://www.faqs.org

Pleasonton, A. (1876). *The Influence of the Blue Ray of the Sunlight and of the Blue Colour of the Sky.* Philadelphia: Claxton, Remsen & Haffelfinger.

Praschak-Rieder, N., Willeit, M. (2003) Treatment of seasonal affective disorders. *Dialogues in Clinical NeuroSciences.* 5(4): 389–398.

Properly Timed Light, Melatonin Lift Winter Depression By Syncing Rhythms. (2006, May 1). *National Institute of Mental Health Science Update.* Retrieved from http://www. nimh.nih.gov

Q & A on Bright Light Therapy. (n.d.). Clinical Chronobiological Group, Columbia-Presbyterian Medical Center. Retrieved from http://www.columbia.edu/~mt12/blt.htm

Rahi, G. (n.d). Positive Ion Poisoning. Department of Chemistry and Physics. Fayetteville State University. http://faculty.uncfsu.edu/grahi/Positive%20Ion%20Poisoning.doc

Rama, E. (2012). Take Back Your City with Paint. *TEDxThesssaloniki.* Retrieved from: http://www.ted.com

Repton, H. (1816). *Fragments on the Theory and Practice of Landscape Gardening.* London: T. Bensley and Son for J Taylor.

Roenneberg, T., Allebrandt, K. Merrow, M. Vetter, C. (2012) Social Jetlag and Obesity. *Current Biology.* doi: 10.1016/j.cub.2012.03.038

Rosenthal, N. (2013) *Winter Blues,* 4th Edition. New York, NY: The Guilford Press.

SAD.org.uk. (2014). *Seasonal Affective Disorder- Information, Advice and Answers from the UK Voluntary Organisation.* Retrieved from http://www.sad.org.uk

Schmidt, C. (2014, July 30). Surgeon General Issues Skin Cancer Warning. *Cable News Network.* Retrieved from http//edition.cnn.com.

Seasonal Affective Disorder (n.d.) In *Wikipedia.* Retrieved July 14, 2014, from http://en.wikipedia.org/wiki/ Seasonal_affective_ disorder

Shipowick, C., Moore, C., Corbett, C., Bindler, R. (2009). Vitamin D and depressive symptoms in women duringthe winter: a pilot study. *Applied Nursing Research* (3):221-5. doi: 10.1016/j.apnr 2007.08.001.

Terman, M., McMahan, I. (2012). *Chronotherapy: Resetting Your Inner Clock to Boost Mood, Alertness, and Quality Sleep.* Penguin: New York, NY.

Terman, M., Terman, J., Macchi, M., Stewart, J.(2005). Controlled trial of bright light and negative air ions for chronic depression. *Psychological Medicine.* 35(7): 945-55.

The Optical Society (OSA). (2014, April 14). *Let the Sun Shine In: Redirecting Sunlight to Urban Alleyways.* Retrieved from www.osa.org.

The Seasonal Affective Disorder Association, UK. (2014). *What is SAD? Symptoms; Treatment.* Retrieved January 11, 2014 from http://www.sada.org.uk

Twohey, M. (2010, March 3). Seasonal affective disorder increasingly a workplace issue. *Los Angeles Times*. Retrieved from http://articles.latimes.com

Vieth, R. (May 1999). Vitamin D supplementation, 25-hydroxyvitamin D concentrations, and safety. *American Journal of Clinical Nutrition*. Retrieved from http://ajcnnutrition.org/

Vitamin D: Fact Sheet for Consumers. (2011). *National Institutes of Health Office of Dietary Supplements*. Retrieved from http://ods.od.nih.gov/

Wang X., Li, C., Xu, J., Hu D., Zhao, Z., Zhang, L. (2013). Air negative ion concentration in different modes of courtyard forests in southern mountainous areas of Jinan, Shan- dong Province of East China. *Ying Yong Sheng Tai Xue Ba*(2): 373-8. Retrieved from http://www.ncbi.nlm.nihgov/

Weir, W. (2012, June 20). Artificial Lighting Poses Health Risks, American Medical Association Asserts Panel Concurs With U Conn Researcher's Report On Adverse Effects, Possible Link To Cancer. *The Hartford Courant*. Retrieved from: http://articles.courant.com/

Wood, B., Rea, M., Plitnick, B., Figueiro, M., (2012). Light level and duration of exposure determine the impact of self-luminous tablets on melatonin suppression. *Applied Ergonomics*. doi: 10.1016/j.apergo. 2012.07.008

Western Regional Climate Center (2002). *Climate of Washington*. Retrieved from http://www.wrcc.dri. edu/narratives/WASHINGTON.htm

'White' light suppresses the body's production of melatonin. (2011, September 12). *Medical Xpress*. Retrieved from http://medicalxpress.com

Williams, T. (2005, June 2). Here Comes the Sun, Redirected. *New York Times*. Retrieved from http://www.nytimes.com.

Yoon, Won, Lee, Jung, Roh. (2014). Occupational noise annoyance linked to depressive symptoms and suicidal ideation: a result from nationwide survey of Korea. PLoS One. doi: 10.1371/journal.pone.0105321

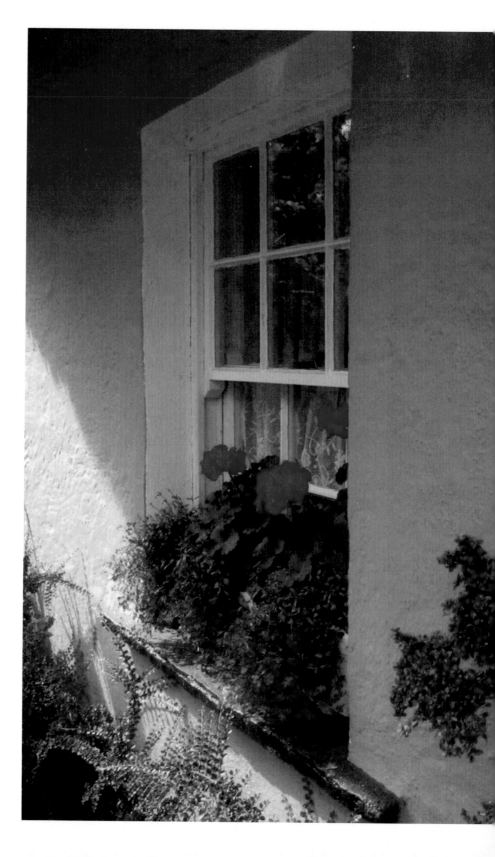

Photos and Illustrations Credits

Photos and Illustrations Credits

All photos, graphs and illustrations provided by the author except for the following:

Cover and pp. 2-3 *Grey skies over Seattle.*
Courtesy of Gordon Hempton.

p. 27 *French dignitary sunbathing in Los Angeles, 1934.*
Associated Press photo.

p. 28 *Sunset.*
Courtesy of Gordon Hempton.

p. 33 *Tuberculous children on the beach at Sea Breeze Hospital, Sea Gate, Coney Island, New York, 1900-1920*
Goldsberry collection of open air schools photographs.
Courtesy of Library of Congress.

p. 35 *Le Chalet, Leysin, Switzerland.*
Courtesy of Fondation Claire Magnin, Résidences médicosociales, Leysin, Switzerland.

p. 36 *Tubercular child on balcony at Sea Breeze Hospital in NY.* Goldsberry collection of open air schools photographs, 1900-1920. Courtesy of Library of Congress.

p. 38 *"Has New Plan To Fight White Plague"* Seattle Daily Times, March 30, 1908.

p. 39 *Children's hospital at Firland Sanatorium, December 9, 1925.* Courtesy of Seattle Municipal Archives

p. 41 (top) *Ballard beach scene, 1890s.* Carl Henry Moen, Courtesy of Lawton Gowey collection.

p. 41 (bottom) *Green Lake beach scene, 1920s.* Courtesy of Seattle Municipal Archives.

p. 43 *Cod liver oil advertisement, March 5, 1922* Seattle Daily Times.

p. 45 *Logging near Cascade Mountains, 1906.* Darius Kinsey. Courtesy of Library of Congress.

p. 46 *Ivanoff Machine Shop in Fremont, 1920s.* Courtesy of Kvichak Marine Industries.

p. 48 *Boeing Aircraft Plant, 1942* Andreas Feininger, Courtesy of Library of Congress

p. 49 *Seattle Street Use Office, 1957.* Courtesy of Seattle Municipal Archives.

p. 54 *Bicyclist on Phinney Ave N.*
Courtesy of Jean Sherrard.

p. 63 (top) *"Cubicle Farm."*
Courtesy of Brian Hendrix

p.63 (bottom) *Downtown Seattle at twilight.*
Courtesy of Bob Warner

p. 70 *People looking out airport window.*
Courtesy of Gordon Hempton.

p. 91 *Group photo at summit of Tiger Mountain.*
Courtesy of Charlie Tiebout

p. 92 *Olympic rainshadow map.*
Courtesy of David Britton.

p. 95 *Seattle rainshadow map.*
Courtesy of Mark Albright.

p. 100 *Valkee light earphones.*
Courtesy of Valkee Oy, Finland.

p. 102 *Computer room at night.*
Courtesy of Jon Ross.

p. 110 *Open Air School #1 and #2 Mary Crane Nursery in Chicago, c. 1913.* Frank P. Burke, Goldsberry Collection of open-air school photographs. Courtesy of Library of Congress.

p. 119 *Brook on Tiger Mountain.*
Courtesy of Seattle Transit Hikers.

p. 141 *Victorian stained glass windows in San Francisco.*
Courtesy of Eric Hunt.

p. 150 *Blooming Monday campaign screen shot.*
Courtesy of Mental Health Research UK.

p. 151 *Woman in yellow dress.*
Courtesy of Rita Hraiz, Rita Hraiz Colour Therapy
Clothing.

p. 159 *Relaxation room at Frey's Hotel in Stockholm, Sweden.*
Courtesy of Frey's Hotel.

p. 161 *Light therapy room at Housing for the Elderly at
Enebacken in Österåker, Sweden.*
Courtesy of Henrik Sellin

p. 163 *Mobile light cafe in Sweden.*
Courtesy of Christina Pohlen.

p. 165 *Indirect indoor solar illumination.*
Courtesy of Parans Solar Lighting.

p. 166 *Heliostats.*
Courtesy of Nikola Berger.

p. 167 *Illumination of NYC courtyard from heliostats.*
Courtesy of John Hill.

p. 169 *The delights of an attached conservatory.*
H. Repton and J.A. Repton, Fragments on the Theory and
Practice of Landscape Gardening, 1816.

p. 170 *People's Palace and Winter Gardens.*
Courtesy of Thomas Nugent.

p. 175 (bottom) *Rendering of proposed atrium in Hveragerdi,
Iceland.* Courtesy of ASK Architects, Reykjavik.

p. 181 *US GSA Central South Building in Seattle.*
Benjamin Benschneider. Courtesy of ZGF Architects LLP.

p. 182 *Rendering of domes - new Amazon headquarters .*
Courtesy of NBBJ.

pp. 187-188 *Boreal© project in Nantes, France.*
Courtesy of Tetrarc Architects, France

p. 191 *Naturhus in Sweden.*
Courtesy of Charles Sacilotto.

p. 199 (bottom) *Allihies, Ireland.*
Courtesy of Dick Keely.

p. 224 *Purple & white flowers.*
Courtesy of Emma Mulanix.

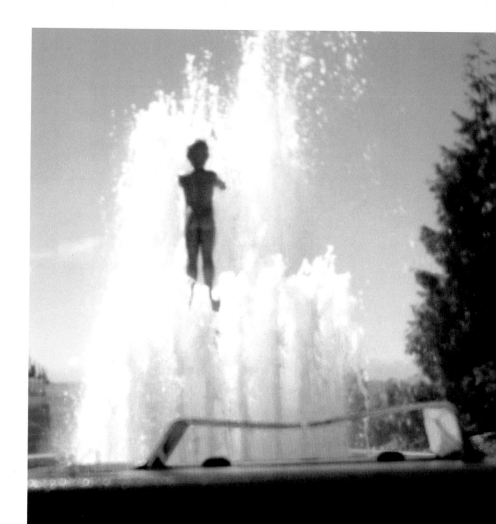

Meters

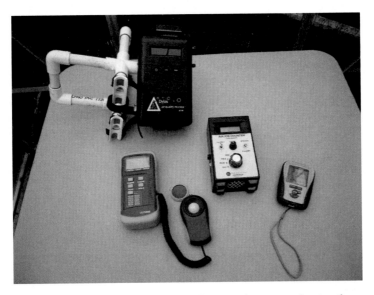

Small hand carried meters helped me to better understand my immediate environment and to become sensitive to changes in it.

Meters

Meters that measure illuminance, barometric pressure and air quality provide specific feedback on what is happening in our immediate environment. Tracking factors such as illuminance levels can help to raise our awareness of changes in the environment that affect our moods and energy levels. Many meters are handheld or can be attached to a bike. The meters used in my research included:

Air Ion Counter: AlphaLab, Inc.
Air Quality Monitor: Dylos Corporation DC1700
Barometer: VWR International VWR® Handheld Digital
Light Meter: Mastech LX1330B Digital Light Meter

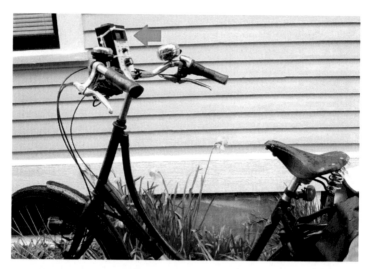

Mounting the air ion meter on my handlebars enabled me to take measurements while riding in the rain. I learned why riding in a heavy rain left me feeling so energized: the many negative ions!

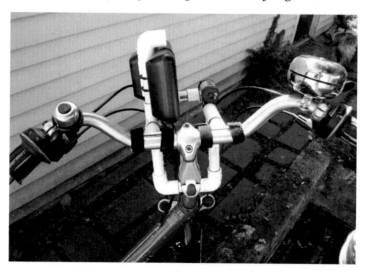

Measuring air quality while bicycling around town has educated me about increased pollution during inversions.

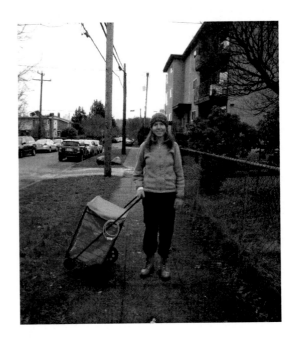

About the Author:

Heather McAuliffe grew up in Seattle. Among her many interests, she enjoys learning about history and health, and tracking light, barometric pressure, negative ions and air quality. Most of all, she enjoys inspiring people and encouraging positive change.

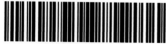

Made in the USA
San Bernardino, CA
16 October 2017